Stories of Dignity within Healthcare:
Research, narratives and theories

Full the full range of M&K Publishing books please visit our website:
www.mkupdate.co.uk

Stories of Dignity within Healthcare:
Research, narratives and theories

Edited by

Oscar Tranvåg, Oddgeir Synnes and Wilfred McSherry

Stories of Dignity within Healthcare: Research, narratives and theories

Oscar Tranvåg, Oddgeir Synnes and Wilfred McSherry

ISBN: 978-1-905539-97-0

First published 2016

British Library Catalogue in Publication Data
A catalogue record for this book is available from the British Library

Notice
Clinical practice and medical knowledge constantly evolve. Standard safety precautions must be followed, but, as knowledge is broadened by research, changes in practice, treatment and drug therapy may become necessary or appropriate. Readers must check the most current product information provided by the manufacturer of each drug to be administered and verify the dosages and correct administration, as well as contraindications. It is the responsibility of the practitioner, utilising the experience and knowledge of the patient, to determine dosages and the best treatment for each individual patient. Any brands mentioned in this book are as examples only and are not endorsed by the Publisher. Neither the publisher nor the authors assume any liability for any injury and/or damage to persons or property arising from this publication.

Disclaimer
M&K Publishing cannot accept responsibility for the contents of any linked website or online resource. The existence of a link does not imply any endorsement or recommendation of the organisation or the information or views which may be expressed in any linked website or online resource. We cannot guarantee that these links will operate consistently and we have no control over the availability of linked pages.

The Publisher
To contact M&K Publishing write to:
M&K Update Ltd · The Old Bakery · St. John's Street
Keswick · Cumbria CA12 5AS
Tel: 01768 773030 · Fax: 01768 781099
publishing@mkupdate.co.uk
www.mkupdate.co.uk

Designed and typeset by Mary Blood
Printed in Scotland by Bell & Bain, Glasgow

Contents

About the editors

Dr Oscar Tranvåg RN, PMHNP, MSN, PhD specialises in caring science, a research discipline exploring and describing the core attributes of caring. He holds a position as postdoctoral fellow at the University of Bergen and Oslo University Hospital. He also works as associate professor at Bergen University College. He has previously published research in the field of mental health, and in dementia care. In his PhD thesis, he developed an empirical-theoretical model of 'Dignity-preserving care for persons living with dementia'. In addition to teaching, he is engaged in research concerning dignified care for people living with dementia, people living in nursing homes, and individuals who desire to die within the familiar setting of their own home.

Dr Oddgeir Synnes MA, PhD is Director of Centre of Diaconia and Professional Practice and associate professor at VID Specialised University, Oslo, Norway, and associate professor at Molde University College, Norway. Synnes has a background in literature and the humanities, and has worked for many years with creative writing and storytelling in elderly care and in palliative care. His PhD thesis was an analysis of the narratives of terminally ill patients. Synnes' main research interests are in narrative medicine, medical humanities and existential care. He has published books, book chapters and articles on these issues.

Professor Wilfred McSherry PhD, RGN, FRCN was appointed Professor in Dignity of Care for Older People in August 2008. This is a shared appointment between the Faculty of Health Sciences, Staffordshire University, and the Shrewsbury and Telford Hospital NHS Trust (United Kingdom). He is also Part-time Professor at VID Specialized University, Bergen, Norway. He is a founding and executive member of the British Association for the Study of Spirituality (BASS) (http://www.basspirituality.org.uk/about-us/). Wilf is a Principal Fellow of the Higher Education Academy and in 2012 he was made a Fellow of the Royal College of Nursing for his unique contribution to nursing in the areas of spirituality and dignity.

About the contributors

Professor Lesley Baillie PhD, MSc, BA(Hons), RNT, RGN is the Florence Nightingale Foundation Chair of Clinical Nursing Practice at London South Bank University and University College London Hospitals NHS Foundation Trust. Lesley's background is in acute hospital care and she worked in healthcare education for many years, combining her university role with continuing clinical practice. Lesley has published in a range of academic and professional journals, particularly on the topic of dignity in care, and she is on the editorial board for *Nurse Researcher*. Her publications include an edited book *Dignity in Healthcare* and a co-authored book *Professional Values in Nursing*. Lesley has a particular interest in quality care, dignity for older people and improving care for people living with dementia.

Professor António Barbosa da Silva BA, BTheol, TheolDr graduated from the University of Uppsala in 1982. He was born on the Cape Verde Islands in 1944. From 1993 to 1995 he worked as an adjunct Professor of Philosophy of Sciences and Health Care Ethics at the Nordic School of Public Health, Gothenburg, Sweden. Since 1995, he has been Professor of Philosophy of Sciences, Ethics, Mental Health and Systematic Theology in Norway.

Dr Sigrunn Drageset, Nurse anesthetist, MSN, PhD is associate professor at the Faculty of Health and Social Sciences, Bergen University College, and VID Specialized University, Bergen, Norway. In her doctoral thesis she focused on psychological distress, coping and social support in the diagnostic and preoperative phase, using mixed methods, quantitative and qualitative approaches in sequence. The participants were also interviewed one and ten years post-surgery in a follow-up study.

Dr Sidsel Ellingsen, Nurse anesthetist, MSN, PhD is an associate professor and program coordinator for Postgraduate Education in Palliative Care, VID Specialized University. In her doctoral thesis she focused on the experience of living with severe incurable disease and receiving palliative care.

Assistant Professor Elin Overaa Eriksen, MSN, RN is a university college lecturer and teaches a one-year postgraduate course in oncology nursing (a 60 international credits post-BA programme) at VID Specialized University, Bergen, Norway. She is also an experienced genetic counsellor at the Center for Medical Genetics at Haukeland University Hospital. Eriksen has also worked with cancer patients for several years.

Professor Arthur W. Frank, PhD is Professor Emeritus at the University of Calgary, Canada, a member of the core faculty of the Center for Narrative Practice, Boston, USA, and a professor at VID Specialised University, Norway. His career has focused on representing the voices of ill people, beginning with his own memoir of critical illnesses *At the Will of the Body* (1991, 2002). His book *The Wounded Storyteller* (1995, 2013) describes the narrative forms that illness stories take and argues that it is morally imperative to witness such stories. His current work concerns narrative practices in therapy, bioethics, healthcare. He is an elected Fellow of the Royal Society of Canada. He is the recipient of the 2016 Lifetime Achievement Award from the Canadian Bioethics Association.

Mrs Karen Grimwood is a Senior Lecturer in Community and Childhood Studies in the School of Health and Social Care, Teesside University, Middlesbrough, England, United Kingdom. Karen has facilitated teams in their quest for excellence in practice and has undertaken several independent external reviews.

Associate Professor Britt Øvrebø Haugland, RN, BSc, MPhil has a background in nursing, social science, theology, management and art. She has held different positions within nursing education – as assistant and associate professor and she was for many years Head of Nursing Education at Betanien University College, in Bergen. She currently she holds the position of international coordinator and associate professor at VID Specialized University, Bergen, Norway. Her main interest, as a nurse, educator and leader, has been to facilitate the individual in promoting their dignity and using their resources.

Robert Dean Luke, from the Nursing Care Section at Fjell Municipality in Norway, has a master's in health science from the University of Bergen, and works in reminiscence-based dementia care. He has published research exploring the environmental reminiscence approach (ERA) to dementia care, and works as a freelance English language consultant on nursing science books and articles.

Associate Professor Marie Kvamme Mæland, Cand Polit, Nursing Science, RN studied at the University of Bergen. Kvamme Mæland is associate professor (first lecturer) at VID Specialised University, Betanien Campus, Bergen, Norway. She teaches a course in oncology nursing (a 60 international credits post-BA programme). Kvamme Mæland has worked with cancer patients for several years. She also has several years of experience as a genetic counsellor working with cancer patients.

Dr Elaine Maxwell PhD, MSc, BA(Hons), RGN, RN is Principal Lecturer in Leadership at London South Bank University and Non-Executive Director at Basildon and Thurrock University Hospitals NHS Foundation Trust. Elaine is also a Trustee of the Florence Nightingale Foundation and a member of the Editorial Board of the *Journal of Research in Nursing*. After a number of years as an Executive Director of Nursing in the NHS, in 2011 Elaine was awarded her PhD for a thesis exploring the implementation of work jurisdictions for new nursing roles. Elaine has a particular interest in improving healthcare, especially from a patient safety perspective.

Professor Robert McSherry is a Professor of Nursing and Practice Development in the School of Health and Social Care, Teesside University, Middlesbrough, United Kingdom. Rob's enthusiasm, motivation and passion for the nursing profession are unwavering. With almost thirty years' experience, he continues to support and facilitate teams in the quest for excellence in practice. In December 2010 Rob was awarded a Fellowship to the Faculty of Nursing and Midwifery from the Royal College of Surgeons in Ireland Dublin (FFNMRCSI) for his significant contributions to nursing. He also received a National Teaching Fellowship (NTF) from the Higher Education Academy in 2011 in recognition of his excellence in learning and teaching. Rob is Adjunct Professor at the University of Tasmania, Visiting Professor at Tehran University of Medical Sciences and was previously Visiting Professor at Narh-Bita University, Ghana, and Clinical Associate Professor at the Australian Catholic University, Brisbane, Australia.

Professor Dagfinn Nåden, from Oslo and Akershus University College of Applied Sciences, holds a professorship in nursing science and leads the research group Dignity and Ethics. He also holds a position as docent in caring science at Åbo Academy University in Vasa, Finland. His research focuses, in particular, on the concepts of dignity, confirmation and nursing as art.

Dr Åsa Roxberg PhD studied caring science at the Åbo Academy, Finland and is an associate professor at VID Specialized University, Bergen, Norway; Linneus University, Växjö, Sweden; Mälardalen University, Västerås, Sweden; and Halmstad University, Halmstad, Sweden. The main focus of her research is suffering, consolation, ethics and palliative care. Her research is based on Job in the Old Testament, relating Job's suffering and consolation to the human suffering that occurred during the tsunami catastrophe in 2004.

Dr Nicola Thomas, RGN, BSc (Hons), MA, PhD is a Reader in Kidney Care at London South Bank University, UK. She has spent her whole career working within the renal speciality and has extensive teaching experience in kidney care, research and clinical leadership courses. Her particular research interest is self-management of kidney disease, and she has been involved in two national quality improvement projects in the UK, funded by the Health Foundation. She has a special interest in patient and carer involvement in education and research. In 2015–2017 she is involved in a co-produced research study on shared decision-making, in which patients are interviewing other patients about their dialysis decision. She has been President of the European Dialysis and Transplant Nurses Association/European Renal Care Association (EDTNA/ERCA) and is Editor of the *Journal of Renal Care.*

Assistant Professor Kjersti Samuelsen, RN, MSc (Counselling) is a Registered Nurse with 15 years of nursing practice from a range of different clinical settings, but mostly within emergency medicine and Critical Care Unit. She has also worked in humanitarian aid and as a student supervisor and mentor. She now works as a nurse lecturer at VID Specialized University, Bergen, Norway.

Mr Kevin Stubbings is a Modern Matron for Mental Health Services for Older Persons, Tees, Esk and Wear Valley National Health Service, Foundation Trust, North East England, Hardwick Day Hospital, Sedgefield Community Hospital, Salters Lane, Sedgefield, United Kingdom. Kevin and his team(s) have spent many years engaging with the Excellence in Practice Accreditation Scheme and are advocates of storytelling and person-centred care.

Foreword

Introducing this book is a privilege. It is on a par with introducing a master class on the theme of dignity in care, in which key strands of philosophical scholarship, research and lived experience are brought together. The chapters are written by experts from different disciplines and different countries who clearly care about dignity in care. They care about what dignity is, and what it isn't, and about understanding how we can provide dignity for everyone, all the time.

Those of us who have been engaged in dignity research for some time can be reassured that familiar and well-trodden philosophical and empirical territory will be revisited and reappraised in this book. We can also be excited by new research that stretches our understanding and offers fresh perspectives on dignity, vulnerability, suffering and human flourishing. This book challenges us, then, to engage with old and new philosophical angles on dignity in care. It also requires that we engage meaningfully with the lived experience of care-recipients, care-givers, families and students.

Narratives or stories are a necessary component of dignity practice, research, education and innovation. In *After Virtue: a study in moral theory*, the philosopher Alasdair McIntyre wrote: 'I can only answer the question "what am I to do?" if I can answer the question "of what story or stories do I find myself a part?"'

This book is peppered with many memorable stories – stories that may delight and disturb us; stories that will reassure us and require us to analyse how dignifying care is possible and why undignifying care happens. Readers will remember and learn from the distressing predicament of Lucy Grealy and her friend Ann Patchett (Chapter 2). They are likely to be moved by the experience of care-recipients, such as Sylvia, who asserts 'I want to be who I've always been' (Chapter 3) and by the experiences of Mary (Chapter 4), Peter (Chapter 6) and Delwyn (Chapter 7). Readers may be challenged by Mrs Johnson's negative response to nurse Sarah (Chapter 8). They are also likely to be greatly heartened by the creativity of student nurse, Ann, in her engagement with Mrs Peterson (Chapter 10).

Author Ursula K. Le Guin said: 'We read books to find out who we are. What other people, real or imaginary, do and think and feel … is an essential guide to our understanding of what we ourselves are and may become.'

This book furthers our understanding of dignity in care. The philosophical scholarship and empirical research summarised here might be said to provide us with the 'why', 'what' and 'how' of good care. We are committed to fully respect the intrinsic value and worth of all human beings (the 'why'); we engage with the lived experience captured in dignity research and stories that illuminate human vulnerability (the 'what'); and we practise drawing on research and practical insights that further our understanding of the moral sensitivity required to engage in meaningful care relationships that promote human flourishing (the 'how').

Crucially, this book will encourage us all to take stock of our many care achievements, to understand some of our failings and aspire to improve what we do. It urges us to reflect on the better care-givers and human beings we may become. I am pleased to have the opportunity to recommend this rich resource to you.

Ann Gallagher
Professor of Ethics and Care, International Care Ethics (ICE) Observatory,
University of Surrey

Preface: The necessity of dignity in healthcare

The term 'dignity' is not only relevant to those delivering and receiving healthcare. Dignity is experienced and expressed in the everyday attitudes, beliefs, values, behaviours and actions of people all over the world, living in many diverse societies. Dignity is hard to define because it is a multifaceted, umbrella term, which makes it challenging to precisely articulate its attributes or constituent parts. Dignity has relevance to all human beings.

The word 'dignity' is associated with respect, pride, self-respect, self-esteem, and self-worth. A review of these words suggests a relationship with attitudes and behaviour. Furthermore, they suggest that dignity may be linked with how an individual may feel or be made to feel through actions and behaviours. This implies that dignity may be uniquely interpreted, experienced and influenced by a wide range of individual, social, cultural, ethnic, religious, political, organisational and professional factors. Therefore, what may constitute dignity for one person may be considered a violation for another. However, most people know when they have been treated in a disrespectful or undignified manner – and we all know when dignity is absent.

The exploration of dignity is also nothing new. The Italian Renaissance philosopher Giovanni Pico della Mirandola (1463–1494) and, later, the German moral philosopher Immanuel Kant (1724–1804) both contributed to our understanding of dignity. Within the healthcare context, ethicists, scholars and practitioners have engaged with this concept over many decades in an attempt to unravel its meaning and relevance for human beings, both individually and generally. Dignity can also be extended to the context or environment in which we live, as human beings.

One thing is certainly clear: the word 'dignity' says something very profound about the status, sacredness and uniqueness of each person. This is because dignity is intricately linked to what it means to be human and the way in which human beings should treat and respond to each other. The intimate and integral relationship between dignity and the person gives the concept a spiritual, transcendent status and significance. A person's dignity can be violated or preserved by the actions, behaviours or omissions of another but it can never be destroyed or removed.

Dignity can be preserved or violated at a number of levels. Extrinsically, this may involve events or conditions that are outside the individual's control, such as the environment, or political, economic or social processes. Dignity can also be intrinsically preserved or violated by factors arising within the individual, such as emotions, feelings, instincts and impulses that shape beliefs, values, attitudes and ultimately behaviours, relationships and practices.

Consequently, dignity is fundamental to every single person's life and history. It is interwoven in everyone's life, shaping people's personal and collective stories. It is not something remote or alien but something that exists intimately, within every person. Therefore, every dialogue or interaction between people can potentially influence a person's sense of identity, self-worth and self-esteem; and furthermore this may be influenced by the social or environmental context in which such dialogues and interactions occur.

While dignity has relevance for all humanity, in recent years the concept has gained prominence within the wider healthcare field. There is a growing awareness of the importance of 'dignity in care'. For almost two decades, in England and Wales specifically, there have been a number of reports highlighting institutional failings in healthcare (The Patients Association, 2009, 2010, 2011; DH 2006). Similarly, the Parliamentary and Health Service Ombudsman (2011, 2015) has published reports highlighting failings in compassion and, more recently, end of life care. However, before one starts to remonstrate, judge, criticise or explore issues of poor standards of care, it is important to affirm that there are many healthcare professionals across the globe striving to provide high-quality, dignified and compassionate care, often in very difficult circumstances. Crucially, there is more good care provided than poor care, and this needs to be acknowledged and the contribution of healthcare professionals recognised and valued.

Dignity violations do not only occur in the United Kingdom but in healthcare contexts everywhere. Therefore, any learning that arises from such failings should be shared and disseminated because an individual crisis may have international relevance. Consequently, the most significant care failings reported in recent years are probably those identified by the Healthcare Commission (2009) in the Mid Staffordshire Foundation Trust Hospital, which initially led to the *Francis Inquiry* (2010) and eventually *The Mid Staffordshire NHS Foundation Trust Public Inquiry* (2013). It is alleged that over 400 patients died needlessly because of neglect and poor standards of care. The public inquiry, held in 2013, indicated that the failings could not be attributed to one specific factor but were systemic – involving a wide range of organisational, managerial and leadership cultural issues that affected the quality of care. One of the questions the public inquiry sought to address was how this culture could have been allowed to manifest for so long in the hospital. Despite safeguards, monitoring and scrutiny by a wide range of professional and statutory inspections, this 'uncaring' culture remained undetected.

All the aforementioned reports highlight the importance of preserving the dignity of those receiving care, and those who are providing care, often in very challenging situations. The reports affirm that everyone has a responsibility to promote and preserve the dignity of the person. Importantly, organisations providing services have an obligation to provide good leadership, creating systems, cultures, environments and processes where individuals can report concerns and raise questions without any fear of recrimination. This 'duty of candour' implies a need to listen to and capture the personal narratives and stories of those receiving and providing care because these may provide valuable insights into the quality of care.

Alongside the publication of the aforementioned reports, several high-profile campaigns have been launched by the Department of Health (2006) and other organisations, such as the Royal College of Nursing (2008), to treat people with dignity and respect. A small number of public pressure groups are continually exposing the poor standards of care provided by some healthcare organisations – for example, Dignified Revolution (2009) and Cure the NHS (2015). These pressures, combined with frenzied media reporting, continually draw the public's attentions to the healthcare service's shortcomings and failings, reinforcing the apparent inability of healthcare sectors to meet the fundamental healthcare needs of an expanding and increasingly dependent population. However, providing high-quality healthcare depends on a number of complex variables, including the attitudes, beliefs and practices of individuals, organisations and indeed society as a whole. Therefore, attention must be paid to the cultural and structural aspects of healthcare, which have a significant impact on the delivery of dignified care.

Listening to the media, and reviewing the vast number of damning reports, is enough to strike fear and disgust into anyone's heart; and of course there is no room for prejudice, discrimination, abuse or neglect, in whatever guise it appears. Yet there must also be a sense of balance and proportion. It is easy to be swept away on a tide of revulsion, and indeed revolution, but this emotional reaction needs to be tempered with caution and reality. The media attention and published reports rightly alert the public to some of the shortcomings in the healthcare sectors and point to a violation of dignity. Yet the media does very little to raise awareness of the excellent standards of care provided by most individuals within the healthcare sector. For example, the *National results from the 2014 Inpatient Survey* (Care Quality Commission 2015, p. 37) provides some very useful insights into the public's perceptions of care. In this survey, question 66 asked: 'Overall do you feel you were treated with respect and dignity while you were in the hospital?' The participants answered: 'Yes always' (81%); 'Yes sometimes' (16%); and 'No' (3%). This is a significant achievement but such successes often go unrecognised when they should be acknowledged and celebrated.

This book addresses growing concern (among patients, practitioners, scholars and politicians) about the provision of high-quality care that is compassionate and safe, preserving the dignity of both the recipient and provider of care. The contributors offer an overview of current research and theory regarding dignity and dignity-preserving care, highlighting practical and ethical considerations in various healthcare settings. Furthermore, the book recognises and celebrates the excellent contribution made by many healthcare professionals in providing dignified and compassionate care that is person-centred as well as relationship-centred, and of the highest quality.

The book is divided into two sections: Section I (Introduction and methodology); and Section II (Stories of dignity within the healthcare context). Section I introduces the reader to some of the key concepts and theories of dignity, demonstrating how the use of narrative can offer insight and practical solutions for the delivery of high-quality care. Section II then introduces the reader to stories of dignity from a number of different settings and perspectives, allowing the reader to engage with core elements of dignity, highlighting how dignity can be preserved – even in very demanding and challenging practice situations. (Please note that these stories have been anonymized. This means that they are based on actual events but the details have been modified to avoid individuals being identified.) Critical thinking activities are used to encourage and foster deep reflection and learning. This book will support students of nursing and allied healthcare professions, as well as healthcare professionals working in diverse practice settings, to reflect upon and enhance the quality of their care, ensuring that it is compassionate and dignified at all times, thus helping to restore public confidence.

Oscar Tranvåg, Oddgeir Synnes and *Wilfred McSherry*

References

Care Quality Commission (2015). *National results for the 2014 Inpatient survey.*
http://www.cqc.org.uk/content/inpatient-survey-2014 (accessed 30 November 2015).

Cure the NHS (2015). *Cure the NHS.* http://www.curethenhs.co.uk/ (accessed 25 November 2015).

Dignified Revolution (2009). *A Dignified Revolution.* http://www.dignifiedrevolution.org.uk/ (accessed 25 November 2015).

Department of Health (2006). *About the dignity in care campaign.* http://webarchive.nationalarchives.gov.uk/+/www.dh.gov.uk/en/socialcare/socialcarereform/dignityincare/dh_065407 (accessed 31 October 2015).

Department of Health (2012). *Winterbourne View Hospital: Department of Health review and response.* https://www.gov.uk/government/publications/winterbourne-view-hospital-department-of-health-review-and-response (accessed 31 October 2015).

Healthcare Commission (2009). Investigation into Mid Staffordshire Foundation Trust Commission for Healthcare Audit and Inspection. London: Commission for Healthcare Audit and Inspection.

http://webarchive.nationalarchives.gov.uk/20150407084003/http://www.midstaffspublicinquiry.com/sites/default/files/uploads/vol_3_chapter_23_footnote_2_hcc0015002863.pdf (accessed 13 May 2016).

Mid Staffordshire NHS Foundation Trust Inquiry (2010). *Robert Francis Inquiry report into Mid-Staffordshire NHS Foundation Trust.* http://webarchive.nationalarchives.gov.uk/20130107105354/http://www.dh.gov.uk/en/Publicationsandstatistics/Publications/PublicationsPolicyAndGuidance/DH_113018 (accessed 31 October 2015).

Mid Staffordshire NHS Foundation Trust Public Inquiry (2013). *Report of the Mid Staffordshire NHS Foundation Trust Public Inquiry: Executive Summary.*
http://webarchive.nationalarchives.gov.uk/20150407084003/http://www.midstaffspublicinquiry.com/ (accessed 31 October 2015).

Parliamentary and Health Service Ombudsman (2011). *Care and Compassion? Report of the Health Service Ombudsman on ten investigations into NHS care of older people.* http://www.ombudsman.org.uk/__data/assets/pdf_file/0016/7216/Care-and-Compassion-PHSO-0114web.pdf (accessed 31 October 2015).

Parliamentary and Health Service Ombudsman (2015). Dying without dignity.
http://www.ombudsman.org.uk/reports-and-consultations/reports/health/dying-without-dignity (accessed 31 October 2015).

Patients Association (2009). *Patients... not numbers, People... not statistics.* Middlesex: The Patients Association.

Patients Association (2010). *Listen to patients, Speak up for change.* Middlesex: The Patients Association.

Patients Association (2011). *We've been listening, have you been learning?* Middlesex: The Patients Association.

Royal College of Nursing (2008). *Defending Dignity – challenges and opportunities for nursing.*
https://www2.rcn.org.uk/newsevents/campaigns/dignity/publications_and_resources (accessed 15 June 2016).

Section I
Introduction and methodology

Chapter 1

Understanding dignity: a complex concept at the heart of healthcare

Oscar Tranvåg and Wilfred McSherry

Introduction

The word 'dignity' is derived from the Latin *dignitas* – *dignas* meaning equality and credibility (Eriksson 1994). The word has particular importance when discussed and applied in the context of healthcare. The preservation of human dignity is of vital importance because the converse (dignity violation) may have a detrimental effect on care and the experience of caring. Therefore, all those employed or undertaking undergraduate or postgraduate studies in nursing or any of the allied healthcare professions require a thorough understanding of the concept of dignity. Having a good awareness of this concept is an essential foundation for learning how this phenomenon can be integrated and promoted in diverse care settings.

Jacelon *et al.* (2004, p. 81) affirm the importance of healthcare education when they write: 'We concluded that learning about dignity was an antecedent to behaving with dignity'. Therefore, being an effective nurse or allied healthcare professional means developing a deeper understanding of the concept of dignity, recognising this as an essential foundation for consciously developing dignity-preserving care as a crucial part of daily practice. This book highlights dignity as an essential element in various healthcare contexts. Utilising various perspectives on dignity (formulated by diverse researchers and theorists), all the chapters in this book contribute to increased understanding of dignity as a core, complex concept, which lies at the heart of healthcare.

Words like 'dignity', 'care' and 'compassion' are often conflated and used interchangeably when in reality they are individual or discrete concepts. However, in healthcare they are often considered to be interdependent and synergistic in nature. For example, compassion may be associated with having a profound awareness of another person's suffering and vulnerability, accompanied by the desire to alleviate and relieve it. Therefore, in order to be compassionate, one needs to respect and have a deep sense of the worth and value of the other person. These are important attributes or defining characteristics of dignity.

The word and noun 'care' is a little more contentious to define since its use in healthcare is often associated with providing attention or treatment in order to meet the needs (often deficits) of the individual. Importantly, the word 'care' says nothing about the attitudes, disposition or behaviour of those providing that care, or the manner or quality of the care they provide. It appears that 'care', as used in this context, is concerned with the instrumental, ritualistic tasks of healthcare – it is something that is done to a person. However, the verb 'caring' implies action and appears to be more concerned with the affective domain (that is, the manner in which care is delivered); this includes the healthcare professional's values, attitudes and behaviours.

Caring is often associated with positive adjectives such as 'kind', 'warm-hearted', 'sensitive', 'responsive' and 'sympathetic'. These descriptions, when applied or used with the concept of care, offer an affirmative image of those providing care, while also saying something about their relationship with those in receipt of healthcare. Therefore, based on this brief analysis of the terms, it is important not to conflate concepts such as dignity, care and compassion but appreciate that each of them have different defining characteristics, depending upon the context and situation in which they are used. Furthermore, this analysis helps to explain why these concepts are often used interchangeably by healthcare professionals.

Dignity as a fundamental quality of human existence

Research shows that dignity is a fundamental foundation for quality of life (Manthorpe *et al.* 2010). However, metaphorically speaking, dignity is a phenomenon that is not easily placed under the microscope and defined (Tranvåg, Petersen & Nåden 2013), and there is currently no consensus on the understanding of dignity as a concept (Gallagher 2011). The concept of dignity (both its practical application and its meaning in the caring context) has therefore been criticised for unsatisfactory documentation, vagueness (Billings 2008), and for being useless in the healthcare context (Macklin 2003). Yet prominent nursing researchers, like Ann Gallagher and her colleagues (Gallagher, Li, Wainwright, Rees Jones & Lee 2008; Gallagher, 2011), argue that dignity is a crucial concept in the healthcare context, influencing caregivers' view of humanity and the quality of care. Gallagher *et al.* (2008, p. 3) states that 'being of value or worth because of the presence of some necessary characteristics' seems to be a generally accepted understanding of the concept of dignity. Moreover, dignity is related to the sharing of humanity (Haddock 1996), a fundamental human quality that can be experienced within dignifying human relationships (Gallagher *et al.* 2008).

Dignity as a human right

Several influential international organisations recognise dignity as an essential need, a fundamental right and an inherent quality of every human being. For instance, the United Nations (1948) emphasises that all human beings have an inherent dignity. This understanding is an essential foundation for the *Declaration of Human Rights*. In *Declaration on the Promotion of Patients' Rights in Europe*, the World Health Organization (1994) underscores the importance of reaffirming 'fundamental human rights in healthcare, and in particular to protect the dignity and integrity of the person and to promote respect of the patient as a person' (p. 8). This declaration also documents how 'patients have the right to be treated with dignity in relation to their diagnosis, treatment and care, which should be rendered with respect for their culture and values', including 'the right to humane terminal care and to die in dignity' (p. 13). In the *Code of Ethics for Nurses*, the International Council of Nurses (2012) emphasise how dignity preservation is part of the core of caring.

Understanding perspectives on dignity

In their practice, nurses as well as allied healthcare professionals may have an intuitive understanding of dignity. However, they often lack the in-depth understanding required to manifest dignity in practical care situations. Despite stated intentions to preserve dignity, circumstances can lead to dignity violations in some healthcare contexts. Therefore, professional caregivers should seek to obtain a deeper understanding of the underlying components of dignity. Such insight will better prepare them to identify and resolve practices that violate dignity, and to recognise opportunities to provide dignity-preserving care (Seedhouse & Gallagher 2002).

Due to its vital relevance in healthcare, there has been an increased interest, throughout the last decade, in exploring the essence of dignity in these particular settings. Researchers and theorists from various disciplines have contributed to our current understanding of dignity. This book demonstrates the influence of dignity perspectives in identifying ethical challenges, preventing dignity violation, and promoting dignity preservation in healthcare settings. Some of these influential perspectives will now be briefly outlined.

Dignity within caritative caring

Katie Eriksson (1988, 1994, 1995, 1996, 1998, 2006), is a Finnish-Swedish nurse. Grounded in the tradition of Caring Science, she has developed the Theory of Caritative Caring for the suffering human being. This theory is anchored in Christianity, Renaissance humanistic perspectives, and Pico della Mirandola's famous public discourse 'Oration on the Dignity of Man' (*De hominis dignitate*) of 1486. In Eriksson's theory, the Latin word *caritas* (meaning 'love and charity') forms the fundamental motive for true caring, and the dignity of each human being constitutes the foundation for Caring Science (Eriksson 1988).

Eriksson (1994, 1995, 1996, 1998, 2006; Lindström, Nyström & Zetterlund 2014), and Edlund (1995, 2002; Edlund *et al.* 2013) document how dignity forms a dualistic concept, with an absolute and a relative dignity dimension. *Absolute dignity* is recognised as an inherent, inviolable and unchangeable dimension rooted in human holiness. In other words, absolute dignity is attached to human worth and the human equality of each person, and can therefore never be reduced or abolished. The latter perspective, *relative dignity*, refers to a changeable dimension that is influenced by external factors. Relative dignity is therefore a potentially violable dimension, in which human beings are offended by other people – for example, due to professional caregivers' non-care, or by other extrinsic factors that devalue and/or insult the unique essence of the individual. However, relative dignity can also be promoted through caritative caring, since this approach invites each individual into a caring communion that confirms and upholds the person's sense of honour and worthiness, alleviates suffering related to illness, and prevents suffering related to caregivers' non-care. Non-care involves all forms of dignity violation that occur through devaluing, offensive or indifferent attitudes and actions among professional caregivers (Eriksson 1994).

Absolute dignity and relative dignity are both basic ethical concepts within Eriksson's Theory of Caritative Caring (1994, 1995, 1996, 1998; Lindström *et al.* 2010). Absolute dignity is a crucial aspect of the human spiritual dimension, containing essential values such as responsibility, freedom, rights, pride, nobleness and worthiness, and thus attached to internal ethical awareness of one's own personal dignity, and the dignity of others. Relative dignity, on the other hand, involves the physical dimension, constituted within each individual's personal ethics, manifested in outward personal behaviour and actions (Edlund 1995, 2002; Edlund *et al.* 2013). In Eriksson's Theory of Caritative Caring, the entire notion of dignity has specific relevance to professions who seem to be the custodians of such concepts as care and caring.

Dignity from a nursing perspective

Exploring dignity from a nursing perspective, Gallagher (2004) describes how dignity can be perceived both objectively and subjectively. According to Gallagher (2004), each individual has *objective dignity* purely because they are human. As each person has human worth, each individual possesses objective dignity, regardless of their personal levels of autonomy, dependency, utility, consciousness or ability to reciprocate in human relations. Linked to the notion of human worthiness and common membership of all humans, objective dignity also constitutes the foundation for the human rights of all people.

According to Gallagher (2004), *subjective dignity* is attached to the individual differences and idiosyncrasies of human beings, and is a form of dignity that is bestowed by other people. This dignity is experienced, subjectively, through the thoughts and feelings of the individual, as this form of dignity is maintained or diminished. A person is dignified when there is a match between personal competencies and circumstantial factors. Moreover, subjective dignity involves both a self-regarding value and other-regarding value, including respect for one's own personal dignity as well as respect for the dignity of others. The premise of objective and subjective dignity certainly has relevance for all those providing care in healthcare settings (Gallagher 2004).

The four notions of dignity

Based on his philosophical perspective on medicine and healthcare, Nordenfelt (2004 and Nordenfelt & Edgar 2005) describes dignity as a complex phenomenon involving four notions. Firstly, *dignity as merit* is a dignity-dimension based on formal positions and social rank. Secondly, *dignity as moral stature* is a form of dignity based on personal moral values. Thirdly, *dignity of identity* is founded upon personal autonomy, integrity and self-respect – a dignity-dimension that is also influenced by relationships and interactions with others. These three dignity notions are changeable, and may vary from situation to situation or from time to time. They can therefore be violated and weakened, as well as supported and promoted. These are similar to the relative dignity defined by Eriksson (1995) and the subjective dignity described by Gallagher (2004).

However, Nordenfelt's fourth notion – *dignity of Menschenwürde* – is a universal dimension of human dignity, unchangeable, inviolable and ever present, due to the intrinsic worthiness of each human being. Again, there are similarities with the absolute dignity defined by Eriksson (1995) and objective dignity described by Gallagher (2004), though they have a different ontological foundation. According to Nordenfelt (2003), additional forms of dignity exist in older people (namely *dignity of wisdom* and the highly general *dignity of merit*), both based on the efforts and achievements of longevity and deserving the gratitude and respect of others. The potential for dignity to be violated should certainly concern healthcare professionals, who have a duty of care to ensure that every interaction with patients, carers and the public promotes and uphold the dignity of each person.

The importance of human interactions

From her position within medical sociology, Jacobson (2007, 2009) documents how human interactions have the potential to be dignity encounters. This means that there is a relational interplay among individuals, as well as collective actors/groups, bringing dignity to the fore – in ways that can either violate or promote dignity. Jacobson identifies *human dignity* and *social dignity* as the two main forms. Human dignity is here identified as an inherent quality and value within each human being, a universal quality, simply by virtue of being human. This basic and essential human worthiness can therefore not be quantified, violated or destroyed.

Conversely, social dignity originates through social interactions, and includes *dignity-of-self* and *dignity-in-relation*. Dignity-of-self is perceived as a quality related to self-respect and experience of personal self-worth, which is in turn connected to feelings like confidence and values such as integrity. Dignity-in-relation refers to how respect and worthiness of a person are conveyed through interactions with others, also involving historical sense of dignity related to status or rank. These forms of social dignity are conditional and measurable, and can therefore be violated or promoted (Jacobson 2007, 2009).

Jacobson (2009) identifies confidence, compassion, solidarity, humane circumstances, order and justice as superior conditions for dignity-promoting encounters. In her Grounded theory based dignity taxonomy, Jacobson (2009) documents how the following relational aspects lead to dignity-violation in social interactions: *Rudeness; Indifference; Condescension; Dismissal; Diminishment; Disregard; Contempt; Dependence; Intrusion; Objectification; Restriction; Trickery; Grouping; Labelling; Vilification; Suspicion; Discrimination; Exploitation; Exclusion; Revulsion; Deprivation; Bullying; Assault* and *Abjection*. On the other hand, crucial relational aspects promoting dignity are related to: *Contribution; Discipline; Independence; Accomplishment; Authenticity; Creativity; Enrichment; Transcendence; Restraint; Control; Perseverance; Preparation; Avoidance; Concealment; Resistance; Recognition; Acceptance; Presence; Levelling; Advocacy; Empowerment; Courtesy and Love* (Jacobson 2009). This list of dignity violations and dignity promotions affirms that every single encounter and interaction between two individuals or more is predicated upon the concept of dignity.

Dignity conservation

In their dignity research, Chochinov and colleagues document how dignity is experienced among people nearing the end of life, describing how this may be affected by their understanding of the other person's perception of them (Chochinov *et al.* 2002). Some of the patients reported how they felt they were a burden, while others felt respected in relation to others (Chochinov *et al.* 2006). Crucial to the *Dignity Therapy Approach*, which has been developed by Chochinov and colleagues, is the dignity-conserving repertoire. This consists of dignity promotion and includes aspects such as supporting patients' sense of self-continuity, role preservation, generativity/legacy, pride, hopefulness, autonomy/control, acceptance, resilience/fighting spirit, living in the moment, and having a sense of normalcy as well as upholding spiritual comfort (Chochinov *et al.* 2002). Based on his extensive work, Chochinov (2008, p. 674) affirms that 'dignity means different things to different people'. This indicates a need for further research to identify the crucial actions needed to preserve dignity in seriously ill and dying individuals.

Contemporary understanding: a short summary

Despite their ontological and disciplinary differences, many influential dignity researchers and theorists are united in portraying dignity as a dualistic concept, while utilising unique and contrasting terms such as 'absolute dignity vs. relative dignity' (Eriksson 1994, 1995, 1996, 1998, 2006; Lindström, Lindholm & Zetterlund 2010; Edlund 1995, 2002; Edlund, Lindwall, von Post & Lindström 2013); 'objective dignity vs. subjective dignity' (Gallagher 2004); 'Menschenwürde vs. dignity of identity, dignity of moral stature and dignity of merit' (Nordenfelt 2004); and 'human dignity vs. social dignity' (Jacobson 2007, 2009). These diverse perspectives document how dignity is perceived partially as an inherent and irreducible dimension of each human being, and partially as a subjective and changeable human dimension influenced by external factors. However, some authors (Chochinov *et al.* 2002; Chochinov *et al.* 2006; Chochinov 2008) emphasise the latter perspective, bringing psychosocial, and spiritual aspects to the fore, highlighting how these may influence how dignity is experienced differently among different social groups.

Dignity in healthcare practice

The aforementioned theories provide valuable insights into various elements of healthcare practice that may either preserve or violate human dignity. They affirm the importance of dialogue and creating caring environments and cultures that are safe, welcoming, comfortable, holistic and truly person-centred as well as relationship-centred. Indeed, it could be argued that this should be the primary goal or aim of every healthcare professional, organisation and government department charged with the responsibility of providing care. It therefore seems a little strange that in England there has been a need for the government (DH 2006), in partnership with other professional bodies (RCN 2008), to initiate a campaign specifically championing the preservation of human dignity.

In November 2006, the Department of Health (England) launched a Dignity in Care Campaign. The aim of the campaign was to stimulate a national debate around dignity in care and create a care system where there was zero tolerance of abuse and disrespect for any person (Health and Social Care Advisory Service 2010). This campaign outlined national expectations regarding what care services that respect human dignity should value and promote. The catalyst for the campaign was an increasing number of allegations that many older people were being subjected to poor standards of care and violations of their dignity. In an attempt to address these shortcomings, the dignity in care campaign consisted of two key strategies: the signing up of dignity champions across the full health and social care sector; and the launch of the 10-Point Dignity Challenge (see Table 1.1 below).

Table 1.1 10-Point Dignity Challenge

High-quality care services that respect people's dignity should:	
1	Have a zero tolerance of all forms of *abuse*.
2	Support people with the same *respect* you would want for yourself or a member of your family.
3	Treat each person as an *individual* by offering a personalised service.
4	Enable people to maintain the maximum possible level of *independence, choice* and *control*.
5	*Listen* and *support* people to *express* their needs and wants.
6	Respect people's right to *privacy*.
7	Ensure people feel able to *complain* without *fear* of *retribution*.
8	*Engage* with family members and carers as care *partners*.
9	Assist people to maintain *confidence* and a positive *self-esteem*.
10	Act to *alleviate* people's *loneliness* and *isolation*.

(Adapted from DH 2006.)

At present there are over 74,000 dignity champions registered with the Dignity in Care Campaign (National Dignity Council 2015). The rationale for the dignity champion network is to develop a social movement where like-minded individuals will challenge poor practice and promote care services that restore dignity to its rightful place at the heart of care. However, given the vast number of people who work within the healthcare sectors, this is a very small number, and arguably *everyone* working in this sector should be acting as a dignity champion. The limitations of the Dignity in Care Campaign have been described by McSherry (2010) – for example, as soon as the funding supporting the campaign is no longer available, enthusiasm and fervour can fade and the impact is often limited and short-lived.

Magee, Parsons and Askham (2008, p. 9) assert that 'It is easier to make pronouncements about dignity than to ensure dignified care happens.' This quotation implies that action is required if dignity preservation and conservation are to be embedded in the everyday practices of those working in diverse healthcare settings. Therefore, we must turn to the second strategy of the Dignity in Care Campaign, which called for individuals and organisations to sign up and integrate the 10-Point Dignity Challenge within organisational cultures, values and behaviours.

A review of Table 1.1 reveals that many of the words used in the ten challenges (highlighted in italics) are very similar to Jacobson's (2009) relational and dignity-promoting aspects. The ten challenges lay out expectations that should lead to the development of positive interactions between patients and healthcare professionals. However, the 10-Point

Dignity Challenge does not only apply to those providing healthcare. Importantly, these points also apply to *organisations* that provide care services, indicating how they should support the *dignity of their staff*, ensuring they are also protected from any violation of their dignity. This principle is important because if those who are providing care do not feel supported and valued, how can they be expected to preserve the dignity of those receiving care? Furthermore, the 10-Point Dignity Challenge is also pertinent to those involved in the education of healthcare professionals.

Conclusion

This chapter has provided a broad foundation for understanding the concept of dignity, introducing key terms, concepts and theories that are directly relevant to the art and science of healthcare practice. The theories outlined reveal how important it is that healthcare professionals adopt appropriate attitudes, behaviours and practices that affirm an individual's self-worth, leading to the preservation of human dignity. Furthermore, the theories demonstrate the pivotal role that healthcare professionals can play in creating caring cultures, environments and contexts that nurture and promote human dignity. The chapter also demonstrates that dignity is intricately interwoven in the rich tapestry of a person's life and history. This is important because every single person is in the processes of creating and constructing their own personal dignity narrative or story.

The next chapter discusses the importance of stories, enabling the reader to engage with the diverse narratives presented throughout the book. These narratives show how healthcare professionals, healthcare organisations and educational institutions can play a fundamental role in enabling each individual to construct their own personal narrative, thus preserving their own dignity.

Finally, dignity provides an ethical basis for all human interaction. Being aware of the strengths and limitations of the many theoretical and philosophical perspectives of dignity presented in this chapter is therefore vital. There is also a need to be aware of other fundamental variables that contribute to promoting and preserving dignity in diverse clinical settings, including the perspectives of patients, family caregivers and healthcare professionals. Notwithstanding the substantial research-based knowledge that is now available, dignity is still violated in healthcare settings. We therefore need to place more emphasis on identifying, exploring and describing dignity as it manifests in everyday life for people in need of care. We must also identify how dignifying care may become the central foundation or touchstone of future healthcare practice.

Suggested reading

For more in-depth understanding, you are encouraged to read:

Eriksson, K. (2006). *The suffering human being.* Chicago: Nordic Studies Press. [English translation of Eriksson, K. (1994). Den lidande människan. Stockholm: Liber Förlag.]

Gallagher, A. (2004). Dignity and respect for dignity – two key health professional values: implications for nursing practice. *Nursing Ethics.* **11**(6), 587–99.

Nordenfelt, L. (2004). The varieties of dignity. *Health Care Analysis.* **12**, 69–81.

Jacobson N. (2009). A taxonomy of dignity: a grounded theory study. *BMC International Health and Human Rights.* 9: 3. doi: 10.1186/1472-698X-9-3.

Chochinov, H. M., Hack, T., McClement, S., Kristjanson, L. & Harlos, M. (2002). Dignity in the terminally ill: A developing empirical model. *Social Science & Medicine.* **54**, 433–43.

References

Billings, J.A. (2008). Dignity. *Journal of Palliative Medicine.* **11**(2), 138–39.

Chochinov, H.M. (2008). Dignity. Dignity? Dignity! *Journal of Palliative Medicine.* **11**(5), 674–75.

Chochinov, H.M., Hack, T., McClement, S., Kristjanson, L. & Harlos, M. (2002). Dignity in the terminally ill: A developing empirical model. *Social Science & Medicine.* **54**, 433–43.

Chochinov, H.M., Kristjanson, L.J., Hack, T.F., Hassard, T., McClement, S. & Harlos, M. (2006). Dignity in the terminally ill: Revisited. *Journal of Palliative Medicine.* **9**, 666–72.

Department of Health (DH) (2006). *About the dignity in care campaign.* http://webarchive.nationalarchives.gov.uk/+/www.dh.gov.uk/en/socialcare/socialcarereform/dignityincare/dh_065407 (accessed 19 May 2016).

Edlund, M. (1995) 'Värdighet – en analys av begreppets betydelse och innebörd' ['Dignity – an analysis of the meaning of the concept'] in K. Eriksson (ed.). *Mot en caritativ vårdetik [Towards a caritative caring ethic].* Reports from the Department of Caring Science, nr. 5. Åbo: Åbo Akademi University. pp. 169–85.

Edlund, M. (2002). *Människans värdighet - ett grundbegrepp inom vårdvetenskapen [Human Dignity – a basic caring science concept].* PhD Thesis. Åbo: Åbo Akademi University.

Edlund, M., Lindwall, L., von Post, I. & Lindström, U.Å. (2013). Concept determination of human dignity. *Nursing Ethics.* **20**, 851–60.

Eriksson K. (1988). Vårdvetenskap som disciplin, forsknings – och tillämpningsområde. Rapport 1/1988. (Caring Science as a discipline and area for scientific exploration. Report 1/1988). Institutionen för vårdvetenskap (Departement of Caring Science). Åbo Akademi. 7/2001.

Eriksson, K. (1994). *Den lidande människan [The suffering human being].* Arlöv, Sweden: Liber Utbildning.

Eriksson, K. (1995). 'Mot en caritativ vårdetik' ['Towards a caritative caring ethic'] in K. Eriksson (ed.). *Mot en caritativ vårdetik [Towards a caritative caring ethic].* Reports from the Department of Caring Science 5/1995. Åbo: Åbo Akademi University. pp. 9–40.

Eriksson, K. (1996). 'Om människans värdighet' ['About human dignity'] in I.T. Bjerkreim, J. Mathisen & R. Nord (eds). *Visjon, viten og virke. Festskrift til sykepleieren Kjellaug Lerheim, 70 år [Vision, knowledge and influence. Festschrift for the nurse Kjellaug Lerheim, 70 years].* Oslo: Universitetsforlaget. pp. 79–86.

Eriksson, K. (1998). 'Människans värdighet, lidande och lidandets ethos' ['Human dignity, suffering and the ethos of suffering'] in The Finnish Association for Mental Health (ed.). *Suomen Mielenterveysseura, Tuhkaa ja linnunrata. Henkisyys Mielenterveystyössä [Ashes and the Milky Way: Spirituality in mental health care nursing].* Helsinki: Suomen Mielenterveysseura, SMS-Julkaisut. pp. 67–82.

Eriksson, K. (2006). *The suffering human being.* Chicago: Nordic Studies Press. [English translation of Eriksson, K. (1994). *Den lidande människan.* Stockholm: Liber Förlag].

Gallagher, A. (2004). Dignity and respect for dignity – two key health professional values: implications for nursing practice. *Nursing Ethics.* **11**(6), 587–99.

Gallagher, A. (2011). Editorial: What do we know about dignity in care? *Nursing Ethics.* **18**(4), 471–73.

Gallagher, A., Li, S., Wainwright, P., Rees Jones, I. & Lee, D. (2008). Dignity in the care of older people – a review of the theoretical and empirical literature. *BMC Nursing.* **7**, 11.

Haddock, J. (1996). Towards a further clarification of the concept 'dignity'. *Journal of Advanced Nursing.* **24**(5), 924–31.

Health and Social Care Advisory Service (2010). *Dignity Through Action Workshop 3: The Dignity Challenges.* http://www.dignityincare.org.uk/Resources/resource/?cid=7544 (accessed 19 May 2016).

International Council for Nurses (2012). *The ICN Code of Ethics for Nurses.* http://www.icn.ch/images/stories/documents/about/icncode_english.pdf (accessed 19 May 2016).

Jacelon, C.S., Connelly, T.W., Brown, R., Proulx, K. & Vo, T. (2004). A concept analysis of dignity for older adults. *Journal of Advanced Nursing.* **48**(1), 76–83.

Jacobson, N. (2007). Dignity and health: a review. *Social Science & Medicine.* **64**, 292–302.

Jacobson N. (2009). A taxonomy of dignity: a grounded theory study. *BMC International Health and Human Rights.* **9**, 3. doi: 10.1186/1472-698X-9-3.

Lindström, U.Å., Nyström, L.L. & Zetterlund, J.E. (2014). 'Katie Eriksson: Theory of Caritative Caring' in M.R. Alligood (ed). *Nursing theorists and their work.* 8th edn. (This chapter was first published in the 6th edn, 2006). St. Louis, Missouri: Mosby Elsevier. pp. 171–201.

Macklin, R. (2003). Dignity is a useless concept. *British Medical Journal.* **327**(7429), 1419–20.

Magee, H., Parsons, S. & Askham, J. (2008). *Measuring Dignity in Care for Older People. A research report for Help the Aged.* London: Help The Aged.

Manthorpe, J., Iliffe, S., Samsi, K., Cole, L., Goodman, C., Drennan, V. & Warner, J. (2010). Dementia, dignity and quality of life: Nursing practice and its dilemmas. *International Journal of Older People Nursing.* **5**, 235–44.

McSherry W. (2010). Dignity in care: meanings, myths and the reality of making it work in practice. *Nursing Times.* **106**(40), 20–23.

National Dignity Council (2015). *Dignity in Care Network.* http://www.dignityincare.org.uk/ (accessed 25 July 2016).

Nordenfelt, L. (2003). Dignity and the care of the elderly. *Medicine, Health Care and Philosophy.* **6**, 103–10.

Nordenfelt, L. (2004). The varieties of dignity. *Health Care Analysis.* **12**, 69–81.

Nordenfelt, L. & Edgar, A. (2005). The four notions of dignity. *Quality in Ageing.* **6**(1), 17–21.

Royal College of Nursing (RCN) (2008). *Defending Dignity – challenges and opportunities for nursing.* https://www2.rcn.org.uk/newsevents/campaigns/dignity/publications_and_resources (accessed 15 June 2016).

Seedhouse, D. & Gallagher, A. (2002). Undignifying institutions. *Journal of Medical Ethics.* **28**(6), 368–72.

Tranvåg, O., Petersen, K. A. & Nåden, D. (2013) Dignity-preserving dementia care: A metasynthesis. *Nursing Ethics.* **20**(8), 861–80.

United Nations (1948). *The Universal Declaration of Human Rights.* http://www.un.org/en/universal-declaration-human-rights/index.html (accessed 19 May 2016).

World Health Organization (1994). *A Declaration on the Promotion of Patients' Rights in Europe.* Amsterdam. http://www.who.int/genomics/public/eu_declaration1994.pdf (Accessed 19 May 2016).

Chapter 2

Dignity and narrative: moral intuitions and contested claims

Arthur W. Frank and Oddgeir Synnes

Introduction

Dignity is valued. To maintain one's dignity is praiseworthy; to violate someone's dignity is culpable. Either way, to speak of dignity is to make a claim: either to sustain one's own dignity, or on behalf of another person's dignity. But what is the content of this claim of dignity? To fill in this content, we humans need stories. Consider the following.

The novelist Ann Patchett (2003), in her memoir of friendship with the writer Lucy Grealy, elaborates the health problems and multiple surgeries that Grealy suffered as a result of the successful treatment for Ewing's sarcoma she had as a child. Grealy became well-known as a result of writing *Autobiography of a Face* (1994), her memoir of childhood illness. Half of Grealy's jaw was surgically removed to treat the cancer, and when she was fully grown, a series of surgeries attempted – unsuccessfully – to rebuild a jaw from bone grafted from various parts of her body.

After one surgery, Patchett finds Grealy still unconscious, lying in a post-operative ward. Her description is graphic and disturbing:

> She looked as if someone had beaten her with a tire iron. Her head was an enormous pumpkin, every feature stretched into someone else. There was blood running out of both sides of her mouth and down her neck, blood running out of her nose. The skin over her eyes had been pulled into shimmering translucence, and her breasts were bare. I was crying then, and I stood beside her and held my hand on her forehead the way she liked. (Patchett 2003, p. 37)

One of us (AF) read this over a decade ago and filed it away. And over the years, I misremembered a significant detail. As I remembered the story, Patchett covered Grealy's breasts. I forgot that she put her hand on Grealy's forehead, but apparently left her breasts uncovered. This mistake of memory reveals a desire for dignity. I wanted to leave the scene with Grealy covered. Leaving her naked was a violation of her dignity.

Patchett, author of multiple best-selling novels that are also critically acclaimed, is a highly skilled storyteller. If she includes the detail of Grealy's uncovered breasts, then that detail matters in how she wants her story to affect the reader. Patchett appeals to readers' moral intuitions about dignity. Those intuitions give the story its effect, and the story then supplements and develops the reader's intuitions. If we want to say what dignity is, we can give various definitions, but these run into the usual problem of definitions: they appeal to words that themselves require definition. Thus, one dictionary defines dignity in terms of *self-respect*, but that only creates another definitional problem. To fill in some affirmative content, eventually, we need a story like the one Patchett tells about Grealy.

Again, Patchett's story depends upon readers already having a moral intuition that when people are vulnerable for them to be left naked is a violation of their dignity – it is not how they would deport themselves if they were consciously in control of their bodies. The story then specifies this intuition; it focuses the initial intuition on an event with characters who act and sensory details that make the action count.

If someone questions either Patchett or a reader who is moved by her story as to why they feel a violation of Grealy's dignity, the only response can be: 'Didn't you hear the story?' This response exemplifies one of Wittgenstein's most famous statements: 'I have simply reached bedrock, and my spade is turned. Then I am inclined to say, "This is what I must do"' (1968, 85e, section 217). If someone else questions why it is what one must do, the only response is to tell another story, and hope that will make matters evident. There is no further appeal.

Wittgenstein's point, and what we mean by a moral intuition, is expanded in the arguments of the philosopher Richard Rorty (1989), writing about people's 'final vocabulary' of value expressions, and the philosopher Charles Taylor (1989), writing about 'hypervalues'. Final vocabularies include expressions of value that can be explained no further; again, one's spade hits bedrock and is turned. Hypervalues are those values that inform secondary, derivative values. Hypervalues are appealed to in defence of these secondary values, but they themselves have no further appeal. Maintaining the bodily modesty of hospital patients is a value; if someone is asked to defend this value, they might appeal to dignity. If they are asked to defend dignity and have no further value to appeal to, that then is a hypervalue.

For Rorty and Taylor, rational debate over values tends to break down among people who do not share the same final vocabulary or hypervalues – such people have difficulty talking to each other, because there is no common ground. Our argument is that people know and express their final vocabularies and hypervalues less often in abstractions and more often in stories they tell. If one person asks another to explain or justify an abstract value, sooner or later that person has to tell a story. But the story will not necessarily convince the questioner, who may have different stories in mind.

Stories are always open to being contested, and so it is with stories that make claims about dignity. Few humans anywhere would say they reject or oppose dignity. But there are varying, even conflicting views about what specifically counts as dignity in a particular setting, what counts as a violation of someone's dignity, and how seriously different violations should be taken. Someone who works in surgical and post-surgical units, hearing Patchett's story, might object that civilians simply do not know, and are better off not knowing, what bodies normally look like immediately after some surgeries. Erving Goffman, in his classic account of how medicine does its work (1961, pp. 330–33), compares medical practice to repair workshops. One advantage of a workshop is that they can take the broken item into a backstage area that is out of the customer's gaze, do what has to be done to fix it, clean it up, and when the item is returned to the customer, it tells no backstage tales. Medicine's disadvantage is that its backstage is populated with patients who remain conscious of what is being done to them and various visitors who see what patients sometimes cannot see. Patchett, visiting Grealy in a backstage area, sees that no one has covered her friend's nakedness. She cries. On some medical accounts, there is nothing to cry over. Patchett's tears are either for Grealy's life as a whole, or else they reflect her medical naiveté.

Here, then, is a controversy between people who would all claim to share the same hypervalue of dignity, but who differ over how that value applies. How much of Grealy's condition, as Patchett not only describes but evokes it, is unavoidable and transitory medical necessity, and at what point is Grealy's treatment a violation of her dignity?

This question is crucial because it specifies what counts as claims of dignity, and how those claims count. What is required for patients to preserve their dignity, and when can healthcare professionals be accused of violating dignity and called to change their behaviour? These questions depend on who tells what stories specifying the contents of dignity, and who is expected to share the evaluative aspect of those stories. An evaluation we, the authors, share – and that we anticipate many if not all readers sharing – when hearing Patchett's story, is that someone could have taken the few seconds it would have required to cover Grealy's breasts. Failure to do that shows a lack of humanity, although with the use of that word, we fall back into the definitional spiral that required a story. So we rephrase: failure to hear Patchett's story and, on subsequent post-surgical occasions, failure to protect patients' modesty opens a moral gap between those who share one response to Patchett's story and those who respond differently.

Goffman's sociological conception of dignity

A conceptualisation of dignity, and claims on behalf of dignity, can be on various grounds: often theological (humans in the image of the divine) or philosophical (most often appealing to Kant). The account in this chapter depends on the sociologist Erving Goffman, who presents an interactional understanding of dignity that we find most useful for applying dignity as a claim with practical consequences in healthcare settings.

Goffman begins his essay 'The Nature of Deference and Demeanor' noting that 'in our urban secular world' a person 'is allotted a kind of sacredness that is displayed and confirmed by symbolic acts' (1967, p. 47). Dignity, on our interpretation of Goffman, comprises both the sense of sacredness afforded to the self, and – because 'sacredness' is another abstraction that requires filling in – the symbolic acts in which sacredness is displayed and given affirmative content.

Goffman proceeds to describe two reciprocal forms of action, deference and demeanour. He defines *demeanour* as: 'that element of the individual's ceremonial behavior typically conveyed through deportment, dress, and bearing, which serves to express to those in his immediate presence that he is a person of certain desirable or undesirable qualities' (1967, p. 77). We understand that as an empirically observable, behavioral definition of dignity, specifying what is meant by the observation that someone 'kept his dignity' in some situation. Alternatively, in the instance of Goffman's 'undesirable qualities', a failure of demeanour precipitates an accusation that someone failed to sustain their dignity. Thus, demeanour comprises the behavioural acts by which people defend their dignity.

Demeanour has its reciprocal action in deference that one person offers to the self of the other. Acts of deference include holding doors as a courtesy, saying 'excuse me', and other gestures of respect. Goffman defines *deference* as 'a symbolic means by which appreciation is regularly conveyed *to* a recipient *of* this recipient' (1967, p. 57). Acts of deference not only recognise the sacredness of another person; they protect that person's dignity. Crucially in healthcare, workers' acts of deference include supporting the demeanour of those who are unable to maintain their own demeanour. For example, covering the nakedness of an unconscious patient. We might call such protective deferential acts *proxy demeanour*. One person acts to sustain the demeanour of someone incapable of doing this for himself or herself.

Deference and demeanour thus function together, as mutually dependent. One person's demeanour calls out the other's deference, and deference is both a resource of sustaining demeanour and an affirmation of demeanour. Unfortunately, the balance between deference and demeanour easily breaks down. Although Goffman does not talk specifically about vulnerability, that is his central concern. Vulnerability is created when persons are deprived of others' deference and of material resources necessary to sustain their demeanour. Goffman's main example is mental hospitals: 'individuals who are the least ready to project a sustainable self are lodged in a milieu where it is practically impossible to do so' (1967, p. 92). A 'sustainable self' here is a self that is displaying a demeanour worthy of others' deference. A milieu that makes it impossible to sustain such a demeanour features 'supervised toileting, hosing down, institutional clothing, forkless and knifeless eating, and so forth' (1967, p. 93). The specifics refer to practices of the 1950s, but a transition to contemporary healthcare institutions is easy to make, bringing us back to Lucy Grealy left naked in a recovery room.

Goffman understands deference and demeanour as moral responsibilities, necessary to maintain the 'kind of sacredness' that the self is afforded in modern societies. To fail in those responsibilities is not only to fail oneself. The failure extends to others in one's immediate presence, and ultimately fails to support an interactive ordering of persons that depends on each both sustaining her or his own demeanour and offering due deference to others. For Goffman, seeing the world as a sociologist, breakdowns of the deference/demeanour system are not individually motivated; but rather, breakdowns are institutionally structured. Institutions support or impede deference and demeanour in their arrangements of physical space, their provision or non-provision of supplies required to maintain demeanour (clothing, grooming aids), and the expectations they set for how persons interact (time limits, terms of address). Dignity becomes most noteworthy when persons manage to support or sustain it despite being in institutional settings that, in Goffman's words quoted earlier, 'make it practically impossible to do so'.

Based on Goffman's distinctions, we can return to the applied ethics of asserting dignity as a claim. In situations where some persons are unable to sustain the demeanour that is the behavioral correlate of dignity, others have a duty to extend deference to include performing acts that assist those who are vulnerable. Lucy Grealy, still unconscious post-surgery, exemplifies vulnerability. Nurses have a responsibility to protect her demeanour in ways she currently is unable to do for herself.

The claim of dignity is the responsibility of those around a vulnerable person to assist that person in maintaining, as closely as possible, the demeanour she or he would maintain if all resources for doing so were available to her or him. While it is true that persons who have the resources to sustain their own demeanour often fail to do so, the duty of *care* is to treat the vulnerable person according to an ideal of demeanour. Again, on this sociological account, this duty is owed not only to the vulnerable other specifically, but to that which any person represents, which is a general principle of the sacredness of the self. While this sociological perspective is only one way to advance claims based on dignity, we propose it as especially useful for thinking about dignity in healthcare, because medical institutions engender vulnerability. These institutions easily lapse into becoming places where the dignity of the self is rendered impossible to maintain in practice.

Four issues of dignity and its violation

With Goffman's distinction between deference and demeanour in mind, we can return to Ann Patchett's story about Lucy Grealy. We understand *dignity* as two complementary duties in mutual relation: a duty of one person to maintain their dignity (acts of demeanour), and a duty of others to offer that person resources necessary to that maintenance (acts of deference). Crucially for healthcare ethics, *duties of deference increase as the vulnerability of the person increases.* That is, as persons become less capable of maintaining their dignity, others become more responsible for assisting them in this maintenance, or what we have called proxy demeanour

To claim a violation of dignity requires identifying persons who either by omission or by commission failed to sustain their own dignity, or else failed to act on someone else's behalf. In the extreme, one person can actively violate the other's dignity. Patchett's story, without saying so explicitly, implies that the absent post-operative nurses violated Grealy's dignity by omitting to cover her nakedness. The story follows a dignity-violation plot: there is an initial vulnerability, someone then fails to assist in sustaining dignity, and there may be a final scene in which the violators are called to account and the moral order of reciprocal deference and demeanour is sustained. Pratchett's story has no such final scene; her tears fill its absence. Other healthcare stories present the complementary plot that describes dignity-preservation. In this plot, an initial vulnerability is remedied by a remedial action that sustains or restores dignity. The force and the effect of both dignity-violation stories and dignity-preservation stories depend on listeners knowing that events could have gone the other way.

We can now offer four summary observations about dignity and ethical claims concerning its violation, from a specifically narrative perspective.

First, dignity as a claim needs stories. Patchett's story shows that in order to make a claim that dignity was violated – or that an exemplary act of dignity preservation occurred – a story like this one needs to be told. The story does not argue abstractly for a concept of dignity; stories are not useful for abstract conceptualisation. Rather, the story presents a series of connected images that are intended to generate a response that is as emotional as it is rational. In response to Patchett's story, some readers will *feel* a sense of offence at how Grealy is treated. It is one thing to speak abstractly of the 'sacredness of the self' as Goffman does. But he needs to tell stories or at least imply imaginable stories that *fill in the content of what counts as dignity*, or sacredness, or other abstractions. Unless evocative stories are told regularly, such abstract words lose their impact; they rust from narrative disuse.

Second, the teller's expected effect of the story is that readers/listeners will respond with an intuitive sense of wrongness at the scene depicted and subsequently call that a violation of Grealy's dignity, among other possible labellings of the scene. Patchett does not speak of dignity; she breaks into tears. As in any story, listeners are called to take the point of view of the narrator, and for that conjoining of perspectives to end, narrators have to be proven unreliable. Sharing the narrator's perspective is the default position, and the case for unreliability bears the burden of proof. So as readers, we share Patchett's emotional response, and that becomes the basis of our ethical judgment.

Dignity is one among a number of words invoked to account for a moral intuition and to make claims for setting things right. *Injustice* would be another such word, or *paternalistic*. As dignity is invoked as the master concept in making Patchett's story actionable, the claim is that post-operative nurses failed in their duty of care for Grealy. They did not necessary fail in their strictly medical care, although that issue is left questionable. The blood coming from Grealy's mouth and nose might have been expected and unavoidable. The failure was in caring for Grealy's dignity. Someone could have put a blanket or gown over her. Or so we are called to believe, as we take up Patchett's perspective as narrator.

It is worth noting that because covering Grealy's nakedness exceeds meeting her medical needs, dignity in this case and in many cases has the quality of being a remainder, that which is left over. Dignity is in one sense – a strictly medical sense – inessential, but in another sense – a humanistic ethical sense – the most important thing.

Third, if someone hears a dignity-violation story and does not have the same moral intuition that a violation has occurred, then a gap opens between those who share that moral intuition and those who do not. A doctor or nurse might see Patchett crying at Grealy's bedside, shrug, and say that if Patchett sticks around the unit for a few days, she will come to view such post-operative scenes as perfectly normal, nothing worth crying over.

When such a gap between moral intuitions opens, the differences are not easily discussed or mediated. As some moral philosophers argue, the first person reacts by believing there is a moral deficiency in the second person who cannot see the situation as the first person does. Mattingly (2014) uses the term *moral incommensurability* to describe such situations. Later in this chapter we will explore how incommensurable different perspectives on dignity seem to be in healthcare work, and how there are different degrees of incommensurability. For now, what matters is the recognition that while stories call on listeners to take the narrator's point of view, the effect of a story's telling can be to solidify a boundary between those who take this point of view and those who reject it.

The fourth point is that the claim of dignity-violation can be made by a third party on behalf of the one whose dignity is violated, and that claim does not depend on the assent of that person. Grealy could wake up and say that it does not bother her that her breasts were left exposed, but in ethical terms, this first-person response would not negate the third-person claim that *human* dignity was violated. If Grealy had no problem with how she was treated, Patchett might feel there was something warped in Grealy's sense of her own dignity, but the first-person perspective does not trump the third-party claim, because the claim is made on behalf of humans universally, and the present person is representative of that larger humanity.

We now present a second story that will help us understand what seem to be the most salient ethical issues for clinical practice: how incommensurable are different reactions to stories of dignity violation, and how might different reactions be mediated?

Dignity in nursing home care

In our research on the initiatory clinical experiences of Norwegian student nurses, we received the following story from a third-year student:

> My first encounter with nursing practice was at a nursing home. It was in my first year and I had no experience with nursing. I was assigned a supervisor in the department who had worked there for many years. My first task this morning, together with my supervisor, was to care for a lady living with dementia. The way she walked into the patient's room made me shrink down to my shoes. She opened the door without knocking, she turned on all the lights, clapped her hands loudly and shouted into the room: 'Now you need to wake up'. She continued by pulling the curtains and opening the window. I was so terribly surprised by how she woke this poor patient. The patient became frightened when we entered. I was thinking about how and what I should do in this situation but ended up doing nothing. Very hard being a student with no experience, the first time in a new practice. One absolutely does not want to be perceived as a know-it-all. But this supervisor has probably gotten into a pattern where she is no longer thinking, only doing. This did something to me. I'll never act like this. Imagine how terrible to be awakened like that.

This story reinforces all four of the points made earlier. First, the story fills in the content of what counts as dignity and when it is violated. The story makes its claim by showing us a violation, not making an abstract argument. Second, the story generates an intuition based on an emotional response. If told well, the story would lead its listeners to hear the supervisor's hand clapping and feel startled, to feel momentarily blinded by sharp light as the curtains are thrown open. The story puts its listeners not only in the position of the student nurse who narrates, but also of the patient who is awakened. Again, if the story is well told, we the listeners do not question the interpretive judgment that the patient is frightened, because we feel frightened. Eliciting that fright is what a story can *do*; it is the story's capacity (Frank 2010).

Third, moral incommensurability might arise, if someone hearing the story takes the perspective of the experienced nurse. A counter-story might be told, narrating the same events, but imagining the patient not being frightened, only confused. A counter-story might expand background features that the student nurse's story omits; for example, the number of patients who must be woken in a limited time period and the need to keep the ward running on schedule. Stories are always open to such revised retellings, and so ethical claims based on stories are always fragile, holding only as securely as interpretive agreement about the story holds.

Fourth, even if the patient was not frightened – or gave no signs of being upset at being woken this way – the student's claim that her dignity was violated would still stand. Conditions including post-surgical unconsciousness or advanced dementia might well suspend or impair conscious awareness of one's own dignity. But claims on behalf of *human* dignity do not depend on the conscious awareness, or even the agreement, of the person being violated. Hospital patients do routinely agree, mostly tacitly but sometimes explicitly, to violations of their dignity. They agree for reasons ranging from indifference, through resignation, to intimidation that is either overt or implied. But that conditional acceptance does not lessen the violation of dignity. It only complicates what should be done in response to that violation.

Narrative deontology

By situating dignity on a narrative foundation, arguing that dignity requires stories be told, we respond to critics who find dignity too vague a concept to be useful. As an abstract concept, dignity will remain endlessly fuzzy at its boundaries. There will always be controversy over whether *dignity* is the most appropriate label to describe what is going wrong in some situation. What counts is not *a priori* specification of the limits of dignity – those limits will always be contestable. What counts is that stories like the two we have presented continue to be told. *Dignity* names the category of those stories, admittedly fuzzy at the boundaries of which stories belong in that category. But fuzzy boundaries or not, the category does not go away.

The problem with *dignity*, in our narrative account, is not vagueness but specificity. Stories make claims of dignity highly specific: here, an uncovered body; there, a rude intrusion into personal space. The significant issues are how far the moral intuition of an ethical violation is shared, and when these intuitions are not shared, are the different reactions truly incommensurable or is there possibility of mediation? The further issue is how far any story asserts a generalisable principle of action. We find ourselves confronting an issue of *narrative deontology*: how far can any story, told about specific actors responding within a specific context, be understood as claiming a generalised duty for other people, elsewhere? How far can any story imply a *rule* in Wittgenstein's sense of being apprehended as something I must do?

We argue that stories do elicit a sense of what must be done – that is their deontological aspect; they generate a sense of duty. Further, we argue that sense of duty requires stories; ultimately it comes from nowhere except stories. This sense of duty, however, extends only as far as people share a moral intuition in response to the story; only as far as the story elicits a shared evaluative feeling about what happened. That local specificity of duty would seem to be a significant limitation of basing ethics on narrative. But in practical ethics, we will argue that locality may not be as much a problem as it first appears.

Dignity contested

We believe the serious and very practical question is not whether claims of dignity are useful or necessary; we are unequivocal that they are. The question is how far conflicts over claims can be mediated. Mattingly's (2014) usage of *moral incommensurability* is important because it is provocative and gives full force to a significant issue. But it risks pushing all cases toward an ideal of consensus that is rarely reached in healthcare.

One of us (AF) once heard a presentation of an ethics case that seemed to represent moral incommensurability. A clinic in the United States diagnosed a foreign graduate student with ovarian cancer; she was recently married but childless. The medical opinion was clear that surgery including a hysterectomy should be performed as quickly as possible. The couple's family insisted that the young woman's priority was to give birth, for the marriage to produce an heir. That was her overriding purpose as a woman. Only after that birth could surgery be considered. The impasse would seem to be moral incommensurability: a radical split between two versions not only of the purpose of medicine, but two versions of the purpose and value of a human life. Those versions are each rooted in their respective communities. Yet this story had, at least provisionally, a happy resolution. The ethics team advised the physicians to back off and let the couple decide. Within a short period of time, they returned for the surgery (Frank 2004, pp. 96–99).

One point of that story is that apparent incommensurabilities are acted upon in unpredictable ways. Participants in contests over dignity claims have more or less space for negotiation, depending on the interpretive communities they have membership in, and what that membership commits them to.

We suggest, as a rough typology of conflicts over dignity claims, three overlapping variations on the forms that conflicts can take.

Dignity trumped

In both the post-surgical story and the nursing-home story, nurses who are accused of violating their patients' dignity either by omission (not covering Grealy as she lies unconscious) or commission (rudely awakening and frightening a patient) might respond as follows. The nurses might acknowledge that how they act is regrettable; in a better world, patients should not be treated this way. They would have some justification for responding along these lines. In the working conditions that are not theirs to change, they are providing the most humane care they can. Post-surgical nurses might say it is far more important for them to monitor patients' vital signs and be alert to post-surgical distress than to worry about having everyone neatly tucked in. Nursing-home nurses might argue (Diamond 1992) that the smooth functioning of the institution requires maintaining a schedule, and if every patient were woken at his or her own preferred tempo, staff would spend the whole day waking patients up.

Healthcare workers labour with a self-consciousness awareness of multiple demands on their time, and they must constantly decide which demands to subordinate to which other demands. One of us (AF) once heard the administrator of a gerontology assessment unit express with the most sincere regret that the pace of the unit's procedures was physically painful to their very elderly patients. But, she added, 'patients die on our waiting list'. Some issues that are claimed to trump dignity do seem like weak excuses for bad care. Other trump considerations, like the need to get to others on the waiting list, are fully honourable. Front-line healthcare workers have to make best use of the resources, including their own time, that they have available. Protesting the need for more resources will not get the present day's work done. But – not everything that does trump maintaining patients' dignity is worth the cost of that violation. How much time would it take to pull a blanket over Grealy; would it destroy the nursing-home schedule to speak in a quieter tone and open the curtains a few seconds more slowly?

In this first type of contest over dignity violation, no one minimises that dignity was violated. What is contested is whether the narrative of dignity-violation is better understood as subsumed within a counter-narrative that prioritises institutional need and resource allocation. Within this latter narrative, dignity is respected but its violations are understood as inevitable.

Lack of empathy

Situations in which other demands on healthcare workers trump their attention to patients' dignity shade into scenes in which the dignity-violation reflects a lack of empathy for the other person. Again, a claim of dignity being violated elicits a counter-story, but now that story refutes either that dignity was violated, or else that dignity counts at all, in this case. Thus to contest the post-surgical story, a counter-story might appeal to Grealy's unconsciousness; she was in no position to know whether she was covered or not, so her dignity was not violated. Or, more extreme, being left naked is a normal part of surgery and patients have implicitly agreed to it as a condition of accepting surgery. To contest the nursing home story, a counter-story might be told in which the patient was either not frightened by how she was woken, or else she would always be frightened upon waking, no matter how much time was taken.

A small library exists of *resentment stories* told by patients who feel dehumanised by medical treatment. The overwhelming volume of these stories raises a fundamental question about healthcare practice: how can some clinicians act like that, even part of the time (Frank 2002)? Many possible answers have been and can be proposed, because the issue is complex and multi-faceted. In their ethnographic study of nursing practice, Janet Rankin and Marie Campbell (2006) present compelling documentation that nurses adjust their own interpretations of patients' needs to match what they have been told are institutional needs. Thus they write about a nurse enforcing a questionably early discharge: 'Her acceptance of the organizational need to accomplish the discharge overrules any nursing judgments that might disrupt the organization. She explained: "But it's already too late, you see. The bed's already booked … And the pressure is on"' (2006, p. 73).

The pressure being on can, initially, lead to the response of dignity trumped. Dignity is still respected, but it is rendered secondary in priority. The nurses described in our two stories – described as absent by Pratchett and as over-bearing by the student nurse – seem to have gone a step further, and that step is anticipated by Rankin and Campbell's emphasis on 'acceptance of the organisational need' as a *de facto* moral guidance system.

Empathy is systematically suspended by repeated, habitual practices of asserting organisational need. Healthcare workers often tell stories depicting patients as either not caring about their dignity (as a result of being too sick or confused), or as having implicitly signed away rights to dignity as a condition of care. These interpretations negate there being any cause for complaint. Even those who do not tell such stories about patients come to believe that their primary responsibility is to maintain the functioning of the organisation. The ethical principle is that maintaining the organisation will ultimately benefit the most patients, most of the time.

This ethic can be described as *institutionally conditioned utilitarianism*. Its rational basis is that healthcare resources are limited, and there is a moral imperative to serve as many as possible. The problem is what kind of individual, face-to-face behaviour becomes justified, and how the habit of those justifications affects both healthcare workers and patients as moral persons. The sense of sacredness about the self is decayed.

Moral incommensurability

People telling stories showing lack of empathy can still express agreement about basic values; the contest is over the applicability of those values in the particular situation. The nurses in both the nursing-home story and the post-surgery story would have no trouble saying they act in accordance with a hospital mission-statement that affirms patient dignity. They have, in the course of their work, developed a particular, practical understanding of what counts as dignity and *when* it counts. Their sense of dignity has been progressively adjusted. Thus, their most generic form of rebuttal to critics is to claim these outsiders do not understand; people who do not do the daily work, with its incessant pace of demands, cannot understand. That argument takes us to the threshold of what can be called moral incommensurability.

Moral incommensurability occurs when each of the counter-stories that contest the applicability of dignity claims is grounded in an interpretive community with its own traditions, coherently inter-related beliefs, and shared practices. People telling these stories become rigidly committed to the interpretive line taken in the story. If the nursing-home nurse were to read the rude-awakening story by the student nurse, it is possible that she might be shocked to see her own behaviour from a different perspective and resolve to change how she acts toward patients. But more likely, she would respond by saying that when the student has worked there longer, she will come to act the same way, because acting that way is how nurses get by in that setting. The crucial factor determining which response the nurse makes seems, to us, to be her collegial support. As the experienced nurse hears the student nurse's story, she imagines the response of those nurses whom she counts as her colleagues, those whose opinion she values, her interpretive community (Mead 1970). She then responds in anticipation of how that group would respond. From a narrative perspective, what counts as *institutional culture* (or more specifically *nursing culture*) is members adjusting their speech or action in anticipation of their colleagues' response. We thus agree with the frequent observation that changing individual behaviour depends on changing institutional culture.

Moral incommensurability is, we emphasise, not individual but collective. Here we reach a significant asymmetry between healthcare institutions and illness experience. Healthcare workers go through considerable training periods during which they acquire professional identities. These identities are then developed and refined in work places that they attend daily. Professionals talk to each other; they exchange stories and share evaluations of what happens in those stories. Even if the specific work group changes, it remains constituted by members who share a common professional culture and who are shaped, over time, by the same organisational necessities. By contrast, people get sick suddenly, families have highly variable experiences dealing with the demands of sickness and healthcare, only some patients find their way to patient support groups, and then only later in the course of the illness. As a result, healthcare workers tell their stories within an interpretive community that supports how those stories evaluate action as ethical. Patients and their families lack those interpretive communities and tell their stories in comparative isolation.

This asymmetry is not news; its recognition is one reason for positions including patient advocates, ombudspersons, ethics consultants, and support groups. The problems include how quickly patients can find those resource people, not whether but how far the resource persons are compromised by institutional employment, and how consistent the support of the resource person can be, given their work demands.

Our point concerning moral incommensurability is that if those accused of violating patients' dignity heard the stories told by people witnessing those violations, the stories by themselves would probably not produce any kind of empathic epiphany. As heard within an interpretive community, the stories would be negated as being either the perspective of ignorant tourists (for example, Patchett) or of neophytes whose training is far from complete (the student nurse). Beyond individual interpretations of stories lies an interpretive community, and that interpretive community is shaped by the healthcare organisation within which it is situated.

Thus we reach our heart of darkness: What remains of individual responsibility in the working world of healthcare?

Conclusion: reasserting dignity

Realism requires maintaining a certain scepticism toward how successfully claims for patient dignity can be asserted in healthcare. We have attempted to delineate the fullest complications that need to be addressed by any proposals for improving attention to dignity. Until these complications are understood, they cannot be addressed. But delineating these complications too well can induce defeatism, and the demoralisation of healthcare workers (Kleinman 1988) is the opposite of our intention. In particular, present-day healthcare workers cannot be held hostage to future institutional reforms and readjustments – including changes to professional cultures – however much those reforms are needed (Frank 2004, pp. 28–29).

The dignity problem for healthcare workers themselves comes to this. One person's display of deference to another person is part of their own demeanour. In showing respect to others, humans show themselves to be worthy of the same respect. When one person honours the dignity of another, that act asserts their own dignity. And vice versa: to violate another's dignity is to lose one's own dignity.

Healthcare workers who walk past Grealy's post-surgical bed and leave her naked lose their own dignity as much as they violate Grealy's dignity. The experienced nursing-home nurse who frightens patients has lost much of her professional and personal dignity. Our first concluding point is thus to underscore the symmetry of dignity. It is always one's own dignity that is at issue when one respects or violates the dignity of someone else (Frank 2004, pp. 28–29).

Our second point is that we believe humans have an ingrained sense of dignity that can be appealed to. Stories are the medium of these appeals. A story can have resonance that makes suffering immediate and undeniable. We understand the nurse who says 'the pressure is on' as morally distressed. She has learned to rationalise acting as she does, and she will act on those rationalisations, but she does not fully accept those rationalisations. A potential for anyone to change on a personal basis – independent of changes in institutional culture – remains.

Finally, Goffman teaches us that deference and demeanour are acted out in small gestures. A facial expression, a tone of voice, a choice of words in addressing someone are all acts of deference that respect the dignity of the other (Komesaroff 1995). Stories, as enactments of events, have the capacity to capture these microethical gestures, give them significance, and model them for others to imitate.

In many healthcare settings, institutionally structured arrangements and directives jeopardise dignity. Goffman remains correct in his assessment of institutions that render dignity 'practically impossible' to maintain, for patients or staff. But Goffman also emphasised how much leeway people manage to find within institutional arrangements. As he wrote: 'Our status is backed by the solid buildings of the world, while our sense of personal identity often resides in the cracks' (1961, p. 320). Stories, unlike institutional mission statements, policy directives and templates, are able to work their way into those cracks and show what people actually do, at their best and at their worst. Stories can create cracks that enlarge the scope of action for those who hear them. Stories may not be able to set people free, but they can show ways toward goals like dignity.

References

Diamond, T. (1992). *Making Gray Gold: Narratives of Nursing Home Care*. Chicago: University of Chicago Press.

Frank, A.W. (2002). 'How Can They Act Like That?' Clinicians and Patients as Characters in Each Other's Stories. *The Hastings Center Report*. **32**(6), 14–22.

Frank, A.W. (2004). *The Renewal of Generosity: Illness, Medicine, and How to Live*. Chicago: University of Chicago Press.

Frank, A.W. (2010). *Letting Stories Breathe: A Socio-narratology*. Chicago: University of Chicago Press.

Goffman, E. (1961). *Asylums: Essays on the social situation of mental patients and other inmates*. Garden City NY: Anchor Books.

Goffman, E. (1967). *Interaction Ritual: Essays on Face-to-Face Behaviour*. Garden City NY: Anchor Books.

Grealy, L. (1994). *Autobiography of a Face*. New York: Houghton Mifflin.

Kleinman, A. (1988). *The Illness Narratives: Suffering, Healing, and the Human Condition*. New York: Basic Books.

Komesaroff, P. (1995). From bioethics to microethics: ethical debate and clinical medicine in P. Komesaroff (ed.) *Troubled Bodies: Critical Perspectives on Postmodernism, Medical Ethics, and the Body*. Durham NC and London: Duke University Press. (pp. 62–86)

Mattingly, C. (2014). *Moral Laboratories*. Berkeley CA: University of California Press.

Mead, G.H. (1970) [1934]. *Mind, Self, and Society*. Chicago: University of Chicago Press.

Patchett, A. (3 March 2003). The Face of Pain. *New York Magazine*. pp. 30–37.

Rankin, J. & Campbell, M. (2006). *Managing to Nurse*. Toronto: University of Toronto Press.

Rorty, R. (1989). *Contingency, Irony, and Solidarity*. Cambridge UK: Cambridge University Press.

Taylor, C. (1989). *Sources of the Self*. Cambridge MA: Harvard University Press.

Wittgenstein, L. (1968) [1953]. *Philosophical Investigations*. New York: Macmillan.

Section II

Stories of dignity within the healthcare context

Chapter 3

Dignity in dementia care

Oscar Tranvåg, Robert Dean Luke and Dagfinn Nåden

Introduction

The purpose of this chapter is to discuss opportunities for nurses and their allied healthcare professional colleagues to provide dignity-preserving care for people living with dementia. Ten studies exploring nurse, allied healthcare professional practice and perceptions in dignity-preserving dementia care were recently synthesised and described by Tranvåg, Petersen and Nåden (2013). The results of this research are presented, followed by a narrative portraying Nurse Don's caring efforts to preserve the dignity of an elderly woman residing at a nursing home. From this narrative, we learn practical approaches for preserving an aging resident's dignity through focusing on specific goals and day-by-day spontaneous caring opportunities.

This narrative is followed by 'Critical thinking activities', which offer the reader dignity-related questions for personal reflection. Finally, theoretical perspectives of 'the suffering human being' and the Theory of Caritative Caring developed by Katie Eriksson, as well as the theoretical perspective of 'absolute versus relative dignity' formulated by Katie Eriksson (1994a) and Margareta Edlund (1995, 2002) (in conjunction with Dagfinn Nåden's theoretical work on 'nursing as an art'), are combined with evidence from research articles on dignity-preserving dementia care. This enables the reader to develop a comprehensive understanding of Nurse Don's activities aimed at preserving dignity in our dementia care narrative.

Learning objectives

This chapter will enable you to:

- Learn how current research describes crucial aspects of dignity-preserving dementia care
- Reflect on how dignity can be preserved in practice, anchored in a narrative portraying professional caregiver efforts in everyday care for an older woman living with dementia
- Gain a theoretical understanding of dignity-preserving care for people living with dementia.

Background

Caring for individuals living with dementia can be challenging. Knowledge of dignity-preserving care should therefore be part of a professional foundation for those working in dementia care. Dementia is a term used to describe a clinical syndrome characterised by progressive and largely irreversible cognitive decline. Many people experiencing dementia retain their positive personality traits and personal attributes. However, as the illness develops, symptoms such as memory loss, language impairment, disorientation, difficulties with activities of daily living, and self-neglect are common (National Institute for Health and Care Excellence & The Social Care Institute for Excellence 2012).

Today, approximately 47.5 million people worldwide live with dementia; and the incidence of the disease increases as people grow older (World Health Organization 2015). Due to our aging population, the incidence of dementia is expected to double by 2030 and more than triple by 2050. The number of people in need of dignifying dementia care will therefore expand exponentially (World Health Organization & Alzheimer's Disease International 2012). In order to meet tomorrow's challenges, dementia care intervention that aims to preserve human dignity must become a national and international priority (Engedal & Haugen 2009; Tranvåg, Petersen & Nåden 2013).

During the past 10 to 15 years, there has been growing interest in this subject. Several studies have explored crucial aspects of dignity-preserving dementia care as perceived and practised by nurses and their associated allied healthcare professionals. Recently, Tranvåg, Petersen and Nåden (2013) conducted a meta-synthesis based on results published in ten scientific studies (Zingmark, Sandman & Norberg 2002; Randers & Mattiasson 2004; Borbasi, Jones, Lockwood *et al.* 2006; Sävenstedt, Sandman & Zingmark 2006; Örulv & Nikku 2007; Rodriquez 2009; Manthorpe, Iliffe, Samsi *et al.* 2010; Jakobsen & Sørlie 2010; Rognstad & Nåden 2011; Rodriquez 2011). This study identified advocating individual autonomy and integrity as the primary foundation for dignity-preserving dementia care, and this is discussed below.

Advocating personal autonomy and integrity

From the professional caregiver's perspective, three separate yet supplementary aspects were reported as prerequisites for advocating resident/patient autonomy and integrity (Tranvåg, Petersen & Nåden 2013):

- Having compassion for the person
- Confirming the person's worthiness and sense of self
- Creating a humane and purposeful environment.

Having compassion for the person (including a genuine interest in the individual human being, professional knowledge and a caring attitude towards the person with dementia) are recognised as crucial qualities for competent professional caregivers (Randers & Mattiasson 2004; Borbasi, Jones, Lockwood *et al.* 2006; Rodriquez 2009; Manthorpe, Iliffe, Samsi *et al.* 2010; Rodriquez 2011). Compassion is seen as an essential prerequisite for advocating personal autonomy and integrity, and therefore a primary foundation for dignity-preserving dementia care (Tranvåg, Petersen & Nåden 2013). Eriksson (2006), describes compassion as suffering alongside another, and portrays it as the source of true caring. Compassion can also be interpreted as sensitivity to the pain and suffering of another. Furthermore, the author reveals how 'this sensitivity or tenderness prepares us to struggle with the suffering of another and attempt to alleviate it' (Eriksson 2006, p. 50), saying that 'compassion is not actually compassion until it has been concretised in action' (Eriksson 2006, p. 51).

Compassion is a fundamental moral dimension of nursing (Von Dietze & Orb 2007), and a worldwide ideal for professional care practices (Hudacek 2008; Ellis-Hill 2011). Professional knowledge concerning the fundamental needs of people living with dementia, supplemented by specific knowledge concerning each individual, provides crucial insights in developing compassion (Tranvåg, Petersen & Nåden, 2013) and foundations for advocating autonomy and integrity in others (Borbasi, Jones, Lockwood *et al.* 2006). This knowledge base is essential for caregiver empathy, and the ability to perceive each person as a unique individual in a unique situation (Randers & Mattiasson 2004). There is also a connection between caregiver knowledge, empathy and understanding – for example, when dealing with the unintentional illness-related behaviour (e.g. verbal and/or physical outbursts or aggression) sometimes observed among those living with dementia (Rodriquez 2009). Empathic insight is essential in order to generate dignity, treating each person with respect and seeing them as worthy of proper care, regardless of their behaviour (Rodriquez 2011).

While an ethic of 'caring about' a person is crucial, an instrumental 'caring for' or 'doing for' is not sufficient as dignity-preserving dementia care (Rodriquez 2011). Establishing a person-centred perspective, caregivers gain new insight into the constituting elements necessary for dignity-experience for each individual (Manthorpe, Iliffe, Samsi *et al.* 2010). Connecting with a person's life-history in a personal way, developing an emotional attachment and sense of 'being like family', can be a crucial dignity-preserving resource (Rodriquez 2011). Supporting the individual in making autonomous choices according to their subjective needs, and maintaining the person's trust and confidence by respecting their need to be in control of their own life, are central aspects of dignifying dementia care (Manthorpe, Iliffe, Samsi *et al.* 2010). Having compassion for each individual is a crucial foundation for promoting caring qualities (Tranvåg, Petersen & Nåden 2013). Self-reflection among professional caregivers, aimed at increased awareness of their own needs and wishes should they be in a similar situation, provides an important foundation for developing compassion for each patient (Manthorpe, Iliffe, Samsi *et al.* 2010).

Confirming the person's worthiness and sense of self involves genuine respect for each individual as a unique human being, with inherent desires or rights to make choices according to their personal subjective needs (Zingmark, Sandman & Norberg 2002; Randers & Mattiasson 2004; Sävenstedt, Sandman & Zingmark 2006; Manthorpe, Iliffe, Samsi *et al.* 2010; Rodriquez 2011). This confirmation of worthiness and sense of self is an essential prerequisite for autonomy and integrity, and therefore a primary foundation for dignity-preserving dementia care. Research indicates that professional caregivers emphasise two sources of dignity among people with dementia: inherent self-respect, founded on feelings of personal worthiness; and respectful recognition and confirmation by others (Tranvåg, Petersen & Nåden 2013).

People living with dementia may suffer gradual loss of identity and personal dignity. In turn, this may lead to depression or social isolation (Pittiglio 2000). However, even individuals with severe dementia may exhibit episodes of lucidity, especially when professional caregivers emphasise person-centred care, affirming individual personal value, while encouraging meaningful expressions of experience (Normann, Asplund & Norberg 1998). Placing emphasis on discovering the personality of each human being generates essential knowledge. Such insight is essential for professional caregivers aiming to preserve an individual's sense of self, while confirming their sense of value (Zingmark, Sandman & Norberg 2002; Manthorpe, Iliffe, Samsi *et al.* 2010), assisting each to retain self-respect and personal status (Manthorpe, Iliffe, Samsi *et al.* 2010). In everyday care, this knowledge encourages the maintenance of the external appearance of each patient or resident – for example, helping them dress and style their hair, as they prefer (Zingmark, Sandman & Norberg 2002). Equally important are daily opportunities for enhancing subjective dignity-related experiences, identified by supporting individuals in a personal way (Manthorpe, Iliffe, Samsi *et al.* 2010).

Including each person in a relational, caring fellowship, and confirming their self-worth through friendly conversation, is crucial to dignified dementia care (Sävenstedt, Sandman & Zingmark 2006). Social interactions can also strengthen personal resources, as settings of this nature stimulate both subjective aspects (such as memory) and relational aspects, through communication and interaction (Randers & Mattiasson 2004). Knowledge of a person's life-history is therefore a valuable source of information for caregivers wishing to stimulate memory and promote choices consistent with each individual's authentic character. Reminiscing about crucial life-projects (Tranvåg, Petersen & Nåden 2014), or getting valuable glimpses of one's own life-history (Randers & Mattiasson 2004; Luke, Petersen & Tranvåg 2013), help confirm individual feelings of human worth and sense of self (Tranvåg, Petersen & Nåden 2013).

Creating a humane and purposeful environment focuses attention on establishing friendly surroundings, which help compensate for dementia-related loss of function among those who reside there. This type of environment is essential in building autonomy and integrity advocacy, and therefore a primary foundation for dignity-preserving dementia care (Tranvåg, Petersen & Nåden 2013). Several studies have shown that professional caregivers of individuals with illness-related memory decline should place more emphasis on environmental factors in dementia care. The contextual milieu and climate (in other words, the atmosphere created by the physical environment) has been identified as a crucial aspect of dignity-preserving care. It is therefore essential to create practical surroundings, based on humanistic principles and values, designed to meet our patients' needs for safety and freedom in everyday life (Zingmark, Sandman & Norberg 2002; Borbasi, Jones, Lockwood *et al.* 2006; Sävenstedt, Sandman & Zingmark 2006; Örulv & Nikku 2007; Manthorpe, Iliffe, Samsi *et al.* 2010; Jakobsen & Sørlie 2010; Rodriquez 2011).

Dementia is associated with reduced quality of life partly because of environmental factors. There is often a gap between environmental demands and personal resources among individuals in the developmental stages of dementia (Holthe 2008). Purposeful environments, which complement activities of interest and meaningful connection with others, may increase their quality of life (Moyle & O'Dwyer 2012). Living environments should be calm and homelike in order to help people with cognitive impairment interpret them more easily (Kielhofner 2009). Establishing purposeful environments means creating surroundings that compensate for dementia-related functional loss. Anchored in humanistic tradition, this perspective focuses on supporting and preserving each individual's remaining resources (Holthe 2008; Kielhofner 2009; Moyle & O'Dwyer 2012). However, there are many examples of institutional dementia care where locked doors are utilised to prevent patients from leaving the facility, getting lost, and so on.

Environmental factors of this nature, leading to loss of patient freedom, are problematic in a caring context, undermining basic human values of personal autonomy and integrity. Research shows that professional caregivers often witness frustration among patients, due to physical hindrances – for example, standing behind locked doors, while expecting freedom of access. In order to preserve personal dignity and reduce loss of freedom experiences, frequent walks in fresh air are encouraged to enhance patients' autonomy and integrity (Jakobsen & Sørlie 2010).

As for assisted-living technology, professional caregivers affirm its value under certain conditions – for instance, if it helps to increase environmental opportunities and enhances patients' personal autonomy and integrity. Electronic tagging, for example, can strengthen personal freedom and promote security for people who like to go for walks but may become confused or lose their sense of direction. It is vital that all assisted-living technology be used to support humanity and dignity and never as a tool to impose dignity-violating surveillance. As an environmental aspect of dignifying care, technological solutions should always be individualised in accordance with individual needs and severity of dementia (Zingmark, Sandman & Norberg 2002).

Balancing individual choices among persons no longer able to make sound decisions, against the duty of making choices on behalf of the person

The complex nature of dignity preservation may lead to essential ethical challenges for healthcare professionals. Professional and ethical paradoxes occur when people living with dementia are unable to meet their own essential needs, and are no longer able to make sound decisions. In some of these situations, advocating patient autonomy may actually compromise patient integrity, violating their personal dignity. From a holistic, human caring perspective, this may lead to conflicts of interest as professional caregivers aim to advocate patient autonomy while simultaneously attempting to preserve individual integrity. Research suggests the importance of balancing the patient's free choice (even among those no longer able to make sound decisions) against the ethical duty to make sound decisions on their behalf on crucial aspects of dignity-preserving dementia care. Professional caregivers confirm their ethical duty to protect patients living with dementia from harmful consequences due to violations of physical integrity or other violations jeopardising human integrity (Tranvåg, Petersen & Nåden 2013). Under delicate circumstances, professional caregivers report using mild persuasion or restraint as necessary interventions aimed at upholding personal integrity and therefore providing a foundation for dignity preservation (Manthorpe, Iliffe, Samsi *et al.* 2010; Jakobsen & Sørlie 2010; Rognstad & Nåden 2011).

Thus, while being trained to promote respect, autonomy and self-determination, professional caregivers experience ethical dilemmas in many settings, especially related to patient needs for hygiene and medication. Although this seems paradoxical, research shows that in certain situations caregivers see *employing persuasion in order to meet the person's essential needs* as a dignifying intervention (Tranvåg, Petersen & Nåden 2013).

Importantly, conscious stimulation of patients' own self-determination and ability to cooperate, complemented by mild persuasion or restraint, are equally crucial dignity-preserving strategies in particular situations (Jakobsen & Sørlie 2010). However, mild persuasion or restraint will not always solve ethical dilemmas. For instance, caregiver attempts may be refused by the person being cared for (Jakobsen & Sørlie 2010; Rognstad & Nåden 2011). Situations of this nature involve a fundamental, ethical challenge for the professional caregiver, who has to decide whether a non-persuadable person (unable to make sound decisions and no longer able to take care of their own personal and essential needs) should be allowed to decide for themselves or not. As an example, professional caregivers may find a patient in their bed full of excrement. In this case, the patient is unable to take care of their own essential needs and lacks the capacity to understand harmful consequences, but the caregiver's attempts to persuade them to accept help, wash and change into clean attire may be declined.

Professional caregivers report problematic and inappropriate situations in the context of professional dignity-preserving care. Paradoxically, in this type of situation mild integrity violation, such as *exerting a certain degree of mild restraint in order to meet the person's essential needs,* has been reported as crucial in given settings (Tranvåg, Petersen & Nåden 2013). However, in cases where professional caregivers emphasise the need for mild persuasion or restraint, respect for vulnerable individuals (and their integrity as whole, indivisible human beings) is a vital foundation for dignity preservation. Interventions of this nature should always be grounded in authorised restraining orders, according to existing legislation. In addition, professional caregivers must remain calm, to avoid increasing patient burden and maintain patient dignity in challenging circumstances (Jakobsen & Sørlie 2010; Rognstad & Nåden 2011).

At times when caregivers experience this type of difficulty in caring for vulnerable patients, 'Sheltering human worth – remembering those who forget' (Tranvåg, Petersen & Nåden 2013) is an overarching principle and metaphor for dignity-preserving dementia care, as perceived and practised by professional caregivers.

Nurse Don's narrative

The following narrative concerns Sylvia, an elderly, retired nurse. After a long career of caring for others, the challenges of Alzheimer's made it necessary for her to enter a nursing home, where Nurse Don was assigned to be her primary caregiver. Ongoing observation and professional insight helped Nurse Don apply the art of nursing towards preserving Sylvia's sense of dignity in everyday life. Here is his story.

A slow-motion caring dance...

Greeting Sylvia for the first time, she seemed very sad as she walked into our nursing home, clutching a mandolin with both hands. The look on her face seemed to imply she might never feel 'at home' again. After helping her unpack, I invited Sylvia to join other residents for lunch. She declined, barely touching the food I brought to her room. Sylvia sat completely still for several hours, just staring out the window. When I asked if she would like to play a tune on her mandolin, Sylvia only shook her head. Enquiring as to her background, she replied, 'We moved from Holland ... after the war ... had no friends, until ... until Martha.' I later learned that Martha was a seventy-year-old neighbour who befriended Sylvia, then only seven. 'We walked together, baked chocolate cake', she continued softly, now with a faint smile on her lips. 'Martha taught me ... to play my mandolin,' her eyes lighting up for the first time as she spoke.

Eventually I learned Sylvia had been a dedicated nurse herself. One of her former colleagues, now residing in another city, visited Sylvia, sharing her colourful past. Caring for the elderly had been 'Sylvia's passion'. Never marrying, she cherished each patient and they truly felt her love and concern. After retirement, she moved back to her family home, caring for her aging mother until she passed away. Living alone, Sylvia was seldom lonely, often inviting friends for fresh baked chocolate cake and a merry tune on her mandolin. They enjoyed visiting museums and art galleries together. Growing older never seemed to bother Sylvia, except for the forgetfulness. Bills went unpaid and sometimes friends waited for her for hours, but Sylvia never showed up. Then one day, unable to find her way home, Sylvia became very anxious, until a passing neighbour escorted her home. Not long thereafter, her doctor confirmed that Sylvia had Alzheimer's.

With most of her family and friends gone, the home nurse began assisting Sylvia with meals and medications, eventually becoming her only contact with humanity. For her safety and wellbeing, her doctor suggested Sylvia move to our facility. My responsibilities include evaluating Sylvia's general health and wellbeing, as well as planning her daily activities. Concern over her needs, interests and values, as well as insight into Sylvia's life-story, have guided my efforts. Careful listening has provided appreciation for her rich life. Sharing time together as she talks about her photographs helps us connect. We rearranged her furniture and hung up favourite photographs as well. Sylvia loved reminiscing. 'See my hospital uniform,' she often giggled, pointing to a large portrait by her bed.

Helping Sylvia establish new friends and avoid social isolation became a major priority. Withdrawn at first, she now eats with our other residents, especially Ruth. On afternoon shifts, we sit together, singing their favourite songs. On sunny days, we take walks, occasionally visiting a local art gallery. When it rains, we bake chocolate cake. Some staff members have other priorities, reporting Sylvia as difficult, repeating her often spoken words: 'I want to be who I've always been.' To help fellow caregivers connect with Sylvia and confirm her unique 'humanity', personal traits and history, 10 minutes of each shift is reserved to assist Sylvia in writing short captions under her photographs. As Sylvia's long-term memory and ability to communicate diminish, this measure will help other caregivers appreciate and understand her better, with the hope of preserving her integrity and personal dignity, as long as possible.

Sylvia is becoming more sceptical now, often declining her medications, eating less, resisting help with personal hygiene. Thankfully, our special connection lives on and I still have her trust. After a recent evening meal, Sylvia asked for her mother. 'Your mother cannot come now, but I'm here for you,' I replied, giving her a gentle hug. Sylvia looked into my eyes and nodded. 'Yes, you're here for me. You're here for me,' she repeated. I asked if she would help me clear the tables, and together we washed and sang until the kitchen was spotless. Afterwards, Sylvia took her medication without protest; a routine fellow caregivers have enjoyed as well.

Sylvia's ability to communicate declining, at bedtime recently, she said simply, 'prayer'. 'Shall we pray, Sylvia?' I asked. 'Our Father,' she replied. Therefore, I began: 'Our Father, who art in Heaven …', and she repeated the Lord's Prayer, line for line. Some of her words unclear, some in Dutch, still, the inner peace in her voice said more than words. After her final 'Amen', Sylvia said very clearly, 'I want to pray every night, but sometimes I forget.' I hung a copy of The Lord's Prayer by her bedside so other caregivers could help Sylvia as well. At present, she recalls but few fond memories from her once colorful past, as we strive each day to preserve her dignity, one challenge at a time.

Critical thinking activities

1. What characterises Nurse Don's care for Sylvia? Write a paragraph in which you reflect on the most important aspects.
2. Did you learn anything new from reading the narrative?
3. Read through the narrative once more, with the following question in mind.
   Which caring or nursing theory, or parts of a theory, would you choose to help interpret this narrative?

Interpretative understanding

The invitation to...

This story includes several components of fundamental care, where the caregiver seems to possess scientific knowledge, skills and competence, while also displaying compassion and other artistic, humanistic elements of nursing. The woman is invited into the nursing home as a worthwhile, dignified human being. The caregiver acts in a creative way, carefully listens to her stories and thereby helps her feel at home. The woman's sadness over moving into the nursing home is met by a caregiver who seems to understand and answers her appeal. From the first moment, his focus is on preserving and promoting the patient's dignity. The story gives the impression of compassionate care, where hand and mind cautiously reach out to a vulnerable human being.

The slow-motion caring dance...

There is a movement in this caring sequence, resembling a slow-motion dance, performed by equal partners. The opening scene tells of one entering a nursing home, sad and 'depressed', seemingly aware of the fact that she can no longer live independently of others. We note how the caregiver meets the woman with respect, nonverbally offering her room and space. He does not attempt to assure her that 'everything will be fine'. Instead, he allows her to experience sadness and suffering, all the while communicating: 'I am here.'

A combination of empathy and creativity makes it possible for the caregiver to see her emotional and spiritual needs, allowing her to confront the pain of a difficult life crisis, while simultaneously finding a way to lift and alleviate her suffering. We comprehend her faint smile and sense a certain degree of satisfaction on her face. This scene characterised excellent practice.

In an effort to become better acquainted, the caregiver eagerly listened as she revealed experiences from her childhood and youth. His genuine engagement assures her there is at least one person at this nursing home who wants what is best for her, someone she can trust. The caring communion created between the two serves as a foundation and point of departure for their journey together.

Magnifying his professional duties, the caregiver assists the woman in writing short, life-history related captions under each photograph in order to make it easier for fellow caregivers to appreciate and connect with her. Further, the caregiver included the woman's new friend in their caring communion. They sang songs, took walks, baked cakes and even visited a local art gallery together, helping her overcome loneliness by bonding with a new friend.

The care given to the woman is at its best and nursing practice is elevated to its rightful position – performed as an art. Promoting and preserving the woman's dignity through caring acts, the caregiver's values and morals run through his tapestry of concern. Relative dignity is often at risk when a person moves into a nursing home. To reduce this risk, the overall goal is supporting her inherent dignity while providing the very best care possible. Here, we witness a harmonious dance where both individuals give and receive, with humble respect for human dignity and integrity at the forefront.

As the woman's illness progresses, care becomes characterised by insight and respect for personal autonomy and freedom. The caregiver does not argue with the woman, but lets her know she has a friend she can trust. This understanding becomes clear in the elderly woman's statement: 'Yes, you're here for me.'

And its fulfilment…

Special vigilance is shown by the caregiver, as intuitiveness and sensitivity are applied in 'reading' the suffering human being, seemingly knowing exactly what to do when the woman says 'Prayer'. We notice a shift in the motion of care, towards a clear, gentle, caring dance, embracing the spiritual domain of human existence. With awe for the woman and her circumstances, she and the caregiver become one in voice and spirit, encircled in a state of wholeness and caring communion. Together they enjoy the quietness and silence; a slow, peaceful, aesthetic scene, where two people see each other in a unique light.

Discussion

It is appropriate to frame this discussion primarily within the caring theory of Eriksson (1992 1994a, 1996, 2006), with specific focus on suffering and dignity, as well as texts regarding nursing as an art, by Nåden (1990, 1998), and Nåden and Eriksson (2000, 2004).

Human beings are viewed as having two forms of dignity: absolute dignity and relative dignity. Absolute dignity, by virtue of being created human, is inalienable. Relative dignity can be influenced by culture and society (Eriksson 1994a, Edlund 1995, 2002).

The first part of the narrative describes an invitation to the woman, displaying a genuine desire to create a mutual relationship and become a companion to the patient.

Invitation and confirmation are of primary concern, a starting point towards establishing a relationship between the nurse and the suffering patient (Lindström 1994; Nåden 1998; Nåden & Eriksson 2000), where the ethical element is contained (Eriksson 1994b), involving a genuine respect for the patient (Randers & Mattiasson 2004). The invitation is a lasting one, conveyed by the caregiver to the patient (Eriksson 1994b); therefore, the invitation and confirmation are not bound to any specific time limit (Nåden & Eriksson 2000), as demonstrated in this story. Confirmation is a matter of encountering the person where they are (Nåden & Sæteren 2009).

Eriksson (1994b) states that it is through invitation that we show our principal attitude, our base values and inherent ethical preparedness towards another. This is in line with Rodriquez' research (2009) concerning compassion. The caregiver's principal attitude and base values express themselves through concrete actions throughout the story, as in helping the woman write short captions under each of her photographs, and are therefore a primary foundation for dignity-preserving dementia care, as stated by Tranvåg *et al.* (2013).

The responsibility of the caregiver reaches beyond the present moment, as an underlying motive of this concrete caring act reveals a future aspiration: sheltering the woman's health and wellbeing as her ability to communicate decreases. The written captions will be helpful not only for the primary caregiver, but for all caregivers, thereby contributing towards two-way interpersonal communication between caregiver and patient, even as her verbal communication declines. In this way, the service towards her helps fulfil the caregiver's mission as a human being as well, thus enabling the caregivers to experience their own absolute dignity (Eriksson 1996, 2006). Such compassion is described by Van Dietze and Orb (2007) as a fundamental, moral dimension of nursing.

What is visualised in this story is the drama of suffering (Eriksson 1994b) in which the caregiver acknowledges and confirms the woman's suffering. The drama of suffering continues into the next act, where the suffering human being is permitted room and space to experience their own suffering (Eriksson 1994b). Permission is portrayed in the moral attitude of this story, as the caregiver allows the woman to decide, while at the same time demonstrating: 'I'm here when you need me.' This demonstrates the crucial importance of genuine moral attitudes and demeanour for preserving human dignity (Nåden & Eriksson 2004).

The caregiver allows the woman space to experience her own suffering and, at the same time, shares in her suffering as appropriate. Knowledge and wisdom are continuous themes in caring for the woman, as we experience her sorrows turning to joy. This coincides with Randers and Mattiasson's (2004) research on dignity, where a person's negative autonomy receives support, thereby respecting their integrity in moving towards a state of wholeness. In different ways, both examples show how creating time and space for a suffering individual can help alleviate their pain.

The third act in the drama of suffering concerns reconciliation as a path to wholeness. A reconciled person enters a renewed communion with others and experiences liberation and freedom to become whole (Eriksson 2006). Even though the woman is progressing in her illness, we witness a person who seems comfortable in her present circumstances, due to the care established by her primary caregiver. Together with fellow caregivers, their caring culture allows the woman to feel more at home. A caring communion seems to be a prerequisite for the patient to reach a state of reconciliation. The woman seems to feel more complete and satisfied even though she suffers from severe dementia. Her suffering becomes part of a new wholeness (Eriksson 1994b) in moments when the woman feels safe, in communion with her primary caregiver who strives to be there for her.

Non-reconciliation occurs when patients feel unaccepted or unconfirmed. Not being reconciled can lead to prolonged or even chronic suffering, in which the suffering becomes more and more deeply ingrained – even a part of one's daily life, a strange and frightening experience (Eriksson 1994b). This does not seem to be the case in this story. Here we observe the caregiver lifting the woman to a level where she trusts him and thereby preserving her relative dignity. The challenge is obtaining wholeness in both suffering and health. Experiencing a caring culture and environment among compassionate caregivers is most important, even crucial, for people with dementia if they are to experience reconciliation, wellbeing and contentment. Such an experience may be expressed as 'coming home' to oneself; or feeling at home in life's present circumstances, despite a progressive illness. From this perspective, feeling 'at home' in life means, understanding the laws of life – that each individual has attained the high human office given them by creation (Eriksson 2006; Nyholm 2015), thereby recognising the absolute dignity of each human being (Eriksson 1996, 2006).

As Tranvåg *et al.* (2014) and Luke *et al.* (2013) suggest, reminiscing about crucial life-projects and meaningful glimpses of personal life-history help confirm an individual's sense of self-worth as a member of the human family. We argue that supporting people with dementia in this way helps reconcile their lives, as they experience even for a moment, a shift in values: from those so important early in life, to values symbolising a level of being and at last becoming, such as holiness and absolute human dignity (Eriksson 1994a, Edlund 1995, 2002). Suffering is still present, yet intermittently alleviated, and personal dignity is promoted. Being a compassionate caregiver in the process of reconciliation therefore means helping a suffering human being towards reuniting spirit, soul and body into a single entity (Nyholm 2015).

According to Eriksson (1994b), a human being is a whole entity, made up of body, soul and spirit. When existing on a level of becoming, the human being is in a state of integral oneness – in such a way that individual parts cannot exist separately from one another. We can see this phenomenon in the last paragraph of the narrative, as the woman and caregiver join together in 'The Lord's Prayer', thereby demonstrating their respect for the core value of holiness and absolute dignity of being human.

The basic structure for all caring is the relationship between the caregiver and the recipient of care, while the ethical element is the way we invite those being cared for into such a relationship (Eriksson 1994b). In the above story, we witness a relationship between a woman and her caregiver, which can be likened to a caring communion – an act of sharing within an intimate relationship with deep understanding (Eriksson 1994b). This relationship is observed throughout the unfolding story; when Sylvia becomes anxious, withdrawn or irritated, the caregiver gently invites her into a caring communion. We sense this communion between the two as a caring dance unfolding at the nursing home, in which caregiver and care recipient become truer to themselves (Eriksson 1994b).

The caregiver takes responsibility for the first steps towards creating a caring communion. The caregiver exists on the level of becoming (fulfilling himself through serving another human being, striving to give the woman the best possible care) – making room for Sylvia's freedom and wholeness, despite her progressing illness. Unselfish love is realised through the caregiver's attitude and generosity, giving the woman his genuine self. It is as if they are walking down the same path together, where love and devotion are part of the journey, as the caregiver helps create room for joy and happiness for his patient, while promoting her dignity. A caring communion is therefore of the utmost importance.

Referring to Løgstrup, Sävenstedt *et al.* (2006) underline that there is genuine communication in a caring relationship and an ethical challenge demanding a response to the needs of those involved. Eriksson claims that all forms of caring are variations of human communion (Eriksson 1992, 1994b). The caregiver creates possibilities for the woman, shaping her life towards wholeness and dignity, while she resides at the nursing home. To use a metaphor: the caring dance takes on a quiet, wavelike motion, softly and cautiously embracing (Nåden 1990), as the tone of the voice, the movement of the hand and the posture of the body equal a quality providing human beings with a sensation of wandering back to their origin in renewed form (Nåden 1998). Thus, caring encounters make it possible for the greatness within a human being to emerge, as human dignity is illuminated and highlighted.

For a caregiver to be prepared to embark on such a journey, in which preserving human dignity is one's goal, competence in both doing and being is required, as well as a willingness 'to give and take in "no-man's-land". As the space in which the encounter takes place does not belong to anyone, except both, no one can control or foresee what will happen in the encounter, at the moment of mutual understanding' (Lindström 1994, pp. 113–14). Choosing such a route for one's journey might provide an appropriate compass, helping one to respect the absolute dignity of individuals living with dementia.

Chapter summary

- Research documents on sheltering human worth as the overarching aspect of dignity-preserving dementia care.

- According to Eriksson and Edlund, absolute dignity is inherent, inalienable, and granted by virtue of being human, while relative dignity relates to experiences of self-worth and human value in relationships with others.

- The narrative and subsequent discussion in this chapter argue that being invited into a caring communion (based on the caregiver's love and devotion) creates room for joy, happiness and the preservation of Sylvia's dignity.

Suggested reading

For more in-depth understanding, you are encouraged to read:

Eriksson, K. (1994). 'Theories of caring as health' in D. Gaut & A. Boykin (eds) *Caring as Healing. Renewal Through Hope.* pp. 3–20. New York: National League for Nursing Press.

Nåden, D. & Eriksson, K. (2004). Understanding the importance of values and moral attitudes in nursing care in preserving human dignity. *Nursing Science Quarterly.* **17**(1), 86–91.

Tranvåg, O., Petersen, K.A. & Nåden, D. (2013). Dignity-preserving dementia care: A metasynthesis. *Nursing Ethics.* **20**(8), 861–80.

References

Borbasi, S., Jones, J., Lockwood, C. & Emden, C. (2006). Health professionals' perspectives of providing care to people with dementia in the acute setting: toward better practice. *Geriatric Nursing.* **27**(5), 300–308.

Edlund, M. (1995). 'Värdighet – en analys av begreppets betydelse och innebörd' ['Dignity – an analysis of the meaning of the concept'] in K. Eriksson (ed.) *Mot en caritativ vårdetik [Towards a caritative caring ethic].* Reports from the Department of Caring Science, nr. 5. Åbo, Finland: Åbo Akademi University. pp. 169–85.

Edlund, M. (2002). *Människans värdighet – ett grundbegrepp inom vårdvetenskapen [Human Dignity – a basic caring science concept].* Doctoral thesis. Åbo, Finland: Åbo Akademi University Press.

Ellis-Hill, C. (2011). Compassion and lifeworld-led care: an emerging field of study. *Journal of Australian Rehabilitation Nurses' Association.* **14**(2), 6–11.

Engedal, K. & Haugen, P. K. (2009). *Demens. Fakta og utfordringer [Dementia. Facts and challenges].* 5th edn. Sem. Nasjonalt kompetansesenter for aldring og helse [National Center for Competence in Aging and Health].

Eriksson, K. (1992). 'Nursing: The Caring Practice "Being There"' in D.A. Gaut (ed.) *The presence of caring in nursing.* New York: National League for Nursing Press. pp. 201–10.

Eriksson, K. (1994a). *Den lidande människan [The suffering human being].* Arlöv, Sweden: Liber Utbildning.

Eriksson, K. (1994b). 'Theories of caring as health' in D. Gaut & A. Boykin (eds) *Caring as Healing. Renewal Through Hope.* New York: National League for Nursing Press. pp. 3–20.

Eriksson, K. (1996). 'Om människans värdighet' ['About human dignity'] in I.T. Bjerkreim, J. Mathisen & R. Nord (eds) *Visjon, viten og virke. Festskrift til sykepleieren Kjellaug Lerheim, 70 år [Vision, knowledge and influence. Festschrift for the nurse Kjellaug Lerheim, 70 years].* Oslo: Universitetsforlaget. pp. 79–86.

Eriksson, K. (2006). *The Suffering Human Being.* Chicago: Nordic Chicago Press.

Holthe, T. (2008). 'Handlingssvikt og tilrettelegging' ['Apraxia and adaptation'] in A.M.M. Rokstad & K.L. Smeby (eds) *Personer med demens: Møte og samhandling [Individuals with dementia: to meet and to cooperate].* Oslo: Akribe. pp. 114–51.

Hudacek, S.S. (2008). Dimensions of caring: a qualitative analysis of nurses' stories. *Journal of Nursing Education.* **47**(3), 124–29.

Jakobsen, R. & Sørlie, V. (2010). Dignity of older people in a nursing home: narratives of care providers. *Nursing Ethics.* **17**(3), 289–300.

Kielhofner, G. (2009). *Conceptual foundation of occupational therapy practice.* 4th edn. Philadelphia, PA: F.A. Davis Company.

Lindström, U.Å. (1994). *Psykiatrisk vårdlära (Textbook in psychiatric care).* Falköping, Sweden: Liber Utbildning AB.

Luke, R.D., Petersen, K.A. & Tranvåg, O. (2013). Dementia care supported by memory stimulating surroundings: Caregiver experience with environmental reminiscence approach. *Nordic Nursing Research.* **4**(3), 269–86.

Manthorpe, J., Iliffe, S., Samsi, K., Cole, L., Goodman, C., Drennan, V. & Warner, J. (2010). Dementia, dignity and quality of life: Nursing practice and its dilemmas. *International Journal of Older People Nursing.* **5**, 235–44.

Moyle, W. & O'Dwyer, S. (2012). Quality of life in people living with dementia in nursing homes. *Current Opinion of Psychiatry.* **25**(6), 480–84.

National Institute for Health and Care Excellence & The Social Care Institute for Excellence (2012). *Supporting people with dementia and their carers in health and social care.*
http://guidance.nice.org.uk/CG42/NICEGuidance/pdf/English (accessed 23 May 2016).

Normann, H. K., Asplund, K. & Norberg, A. (1998). Episodes of lucidity with severe dementia as narrated by formal carers. *Journal of Advanced Nursing.* **28**(6), 1295–1300.

Nyholm, L. (2015). *Urvilja – när livet är människans hem (Will – when life is the home of the human being).* Doctoral thesis. Åbo, Finland: Åbo Akademi University Press.

Nåden, D. (1990). *Sykepleiens kunstdimensjon (The art dimension of nursing).* Oslo: Universitetsforlaget.

Nåden, D. (1998). *Når sykepleie er kunstutøvelse. En undersøkelse av noen nødvendige forutsetninger for sykepleie som kunst (When nursing becomes an art. An inquiry of some necessary prerequisites of nursing as art).* Doctoral thesis. Vasa, Finland: Department of Caring Science, Åbo Akademi University.

Nåden, D. & Eriksson, K. (2000). The phenomenon of confirmation: An aspect of nursing as an art. *International Journal for Human Caring.* **4**(3), 23–28.

Nåden, D. & Eriksson, K. (2004). Understanding the importance of values and moral attitudes in nursing care in preserving human dignity. *Nursing Science Quarterly.* **17**(1), 86–91.

Nåden, D. & Sæteren, B. (2009). To witness the patient's call. Nurses' perceptions of the phenomenon of confirmation in a cancer context. *International Journal for Human Caring.* **13**(3), 47–55.

Örulv, L. & Nikku, N. (2007). Dignity work in dementia care. *Dementia.* **6**(4), 507–24.

Pittiglio, L. (2000). Use of reminiscence therapy among patients with Alzheimer's disease. *Lippincott's Case Management.* **5**(6), 216–20.

Randers, I. & Mattiasson, A.C. (2004). Autonomy and integrity: upholding older adult patients' dignity. *Journal of Advanced Nursing.* **45**(1), 63–71.

Rodriquez, J. (2009). Attributions of agency and the construction of moral order: dementia, death and dignity in nursing-home care. *Social Psychology Quarterly.* **72**(2), 165–79.

Rodriquez J. (2011). 'It's a dignity thing': nursing home care workers' use of emotions. *Sociological Forum* (Randolph N. J.). **26**(2), 265–86.

Rognstad, M.K. & Nåden, D. (2011). Utfordringer og kompetanse i demensomsorgen: Pleieres perspektiv [Challenges and competence in dementia care: caregivers' perspective]. *Nordisk Sygeplejeforskning [Nordic Nursing Research].* **2**(1), 143–55.

Sävenstedt, S., Sandman, P.O. & Zingmark, K. (2006). The duality in using information and communication technology in elder care. *Journal of Advanced Nursing.* **56**(1), 17–25.

Tranvåg, O., Petersen, K.A. & Nåden, D. (2013). Dignity-preserving dementia care: A metasynthesis. *Nursing Ethics.* **20**(8), 861–80.

Tranvåg, O., Petersen, K.A. & Nåden, D. (2014). Crucial dimensions constituting dignity experience in persons living with dementia. *Dementia.* **15**(4) 578–95

Von Dietze, E. & Orb, A. (2000). Compassionate care: a moral dimension of nursing. *Nursing Inquiry.* 7, 166–74.

World Health Organization and Alzheimer's Disease International (2012). *Dementia: a public health priority.*
http://www.who.int/mental_health/publications/dementia_report_2012/en/ (accessed 24 May 2016).

World Health Organization (2015). *Dementia. Fact Sheet March 2015.* http://www.who.int/mediacentre/factsheets/fs362/en/ (accessed 23 July 2016).

Zingmark, K., Sandman, P.O. & Norberg, A. (2002). Promoting a good life among people with Alzheimer's disease. *Journal of Advanced Nursing.* **38**(1), 50–58.

Chapter 4

Dignity, protected by caring in care

Sigrunn Drageset and Sidsel Ellingsen

Introduction

Dignity and care are important in life in general and especially when vulnerability becomes apparent. Human beings are vulnerable. We are born totally helpless, dependent on others to take care of us for our survival. We are always vulnerable, but in the course of our lives health conditions (such as illness) sometimes make our weakness more obvious. However, the *way* an individual is cared for is crucial. It is that that reveals the importance of the concept of dignity and how it is connected to care. A patient's experience of whether or not their dignity is safeguarded is significant in terms of the quality of care received.

This chapter presents a woman's narrative, beginning with the suspicion of cancer and its diagnosis and progressing to the terminal phase, where vulnerability is prominent. Patients affected by cancer experience existential suffering – in addition to treatment-related problems, such as pain, changed physical appearance, anxiety and depression. They go through different phases that need various kinds of attention and care, during which it is important to protect their dignity. By examining this narrative, we focus on the relationship between dignity and care.

We begin with the theoretical background, including Nordenfelt's concepts of dignity and Martinsen's philosophy of caring. Martinsen is particularly concerned about care for patients in vulnerable situations. Martinsen's (2006) theory emphasises *relation, action and morality* in care (Alvsvåg 2010). Nordenfelt and Edgar's (2005) four dimensions of dignity – *universal human dignity, the dignity of merit, the dignity of moral stature* and *the dignity of identity* – are all evident in these aspects of care. Next, we present our narrative, followed by some critical thinking questions. Finally, we discuss the narrative in the light of the theoretical background and relevant literature.

Learning objectives

This chapter will enable you to:

- Apply the theoretical concepts of dignity and care in relation to a patient's history
- Reflect upon how closely the notion of dignity is associated with the concepts of care and caring
- Recognise how dignity provides a basis for the quality of care.

Background

'Dignity' and 'care' are everyday words with great significance for human life. The Global Dignity (2015) organisation argues that dignity revolves around three ideas, as follows:

- We possess inherent dignity by virtue of being human.
- Our human rights involve how we are entitled to be treated/being treated appropriately.
- Our experiences of dignity are affected by how we treat one another; that is, what we can do to strengthen our own and others' dignity.

Dignity may be defined as a concept that relates to basic humanity. Dignity consists of internal and external dimensions, which are common to all humans and at the same time unique to each person, relating to social and cultural aspects (Anderberg *et al.* 2007). In life, especially when it becomes fragile, it is essential that the individual's dignity be protected.

According to Nordenfelt (2004) and Nordenfelt and Edgar (2005), there are four notions of dignity: the universal human dignity, the dignity of merit, the dignity of moral or existential stature, and the dignity of identity. Nordenfelt (2004) describes these four notions in the following manner:

1. *The universal human dignity (Menschenwürde)* does not vary and is associated with being human and with basic human rights. All human beings have the same value, regardless of ethnicity, cultural background, religion and gender. Nobody should be treated with less respect than anyone else.

2. *The dignity of merit* depends on differing degrees of social rank and position. A person may be born with such dignity – for example, a king. Others, such as bishops or doctors, have a special dignity of merit that comes with their position, and this is called the formal dignity of merit. Informal dignity of merit is earned by through people's deeds, for which they deserve respect. Individuals who possess informal dignity of merit might include, for instance, artists and athletes who promote good values.

3. *The dignity of moral stature* is connected to self-respect and an individual's character and deeds that are of value to them. Moral stature is tied to actions that the person knows

are good or bad, through which their self-respect can be enforced, reduced or lost. For example, if nurses feel pressured to act against their own professional convictions over time, their self-respect will be in danger of being destroyed.

4. *The dignity of identity* is linked to the integrity of the subject's body and mind. Nordenfelt (2004) emphasises that this kind of dignity is probably the most important in the context of dignity and illness. The dignity of illness has evolved over time, partly based on how someone has been seen, heard, recognised or ignored by others. It is significant that this kind of dignity can be taken from us by external events, by the acts of other people, as well as by injury and illness.

Defining care and caring

Care and caring are multidimensional concepts that can be described in several ways. These concepts are important in life in general and are not tied to a particular profession but are particularly vital among professionals whose role is to take care of people in vulnerable situations (Ellingsen 2015). According to the Norwegian nurse and philosopher Kari Martinsen (2005), care is a three-dimensional concept consisting of *relation, action* and *morality*. These three dimensions cannot be viewed in isolation, as they are always interwoven with each other. A relation and an action should also always be morally proper. Care not only forms the value base of nursing but is also a fundamental precondition for our lives (Alvsvåg 2010, p. 173).

However, there is a difference between care and caring. We can illustrate this difference with the question: 'What happens when caring is absent in care?' In professional contexts, caring requires not only education and training but also attitudes where the quality of the relationship is shown through practical action (Martinsen, 2003, pp. 21–28). According to Martinsen, caring is primarily relational. We are vulnerable and born completely helpless, and we continue to depend on one another to survive. It follows a universal moral principle that we should take responsibility for one another and for the weak, sick and helpless. The second dimension of care is practice. Without action, care is reduced to sentimentality. The precise nature of the action and how it should be performed will vary according to the particular situation, context, culture and profession, but is always justified by the condition of the needy. An action can be properly conducted and justified, yet be experienced as offensive and humiliating. Morality, which refers to our way of being in the relationship and the manner in which the action is performed, is therefore the third dimension of care.

Mary's story

We now present a narrative describing the pathway from the suspicion of cancer through the diagnostic, curative and palliative phases. The narrative emerged from several in-depth interviews (Drageset *et al.* 2010, 2011, 2012; Ellingsen *et al.* 2013, 2014, 2015). The sample consisted of patients with different types of cancer, but the majority were women with breast cancer. Regarding our narrative, Mary was 56 years old and lived with her husband and one of their three children. She was a nurse in full-time employment and with no previous serious disease. One morning, having returned home exhausted from her night duty at the hospital, she discovered a lump in one breast when she undressed. That morning, her life changed. Every year, 1.7 million people around the world have a similar experience (World Health Organization 2015).

Pre-diagnosis

I found a lump in my breast and thought, what could it be? I immediately thought that this was cancer. It was a terrible experience, one of the worst in my life. It was impossible for me to sleep in spite of my tiredness. I was so upset and worried. All sorts of thoughts were swirling in my head. I made myself a cup of tea and waited for the doctor's office to open, so I could book an appointment with my GP. I got an appointment the same day at one o'clock. It was good to (go) quickly to my GP, but it made me even more nervous as it confirmed that this could be serious. I had not previously met the doctor, but I felt (that) he took me seriously at once. He listened to me and examined my breast and axillaries. He told me straightforwardly that he suspected breast cancer and wanted to refer me to the hospital, to the breast clinic unit for investigation and mammography. The doctor said to me, 'I think you have to wait some days for further investigation at the hospital. If you do not hear anything, you may call them to (know) if you are on their waiting list'. I thought (that he) was a nice doctor; he did exactly what I wanted. I decided not to tell anyone yet. I was afraid to scare my family unnecessarily. However, while waiting, I was not quite myself. I thought about what this could be, and my thoughts occupied most of my attention.

Diagnostic phase

After five days, I got my examination (results). I still hadn't told my husband or anybody else. At the hospital, they (performed a) mammography, (an) ultrasound and (a) core needle biopsy. During the different examinations, I was in and out of the waiting room. The doctor (who) performed the examination had told me right away that I had to be prepared that it could be cancer. I went out to the waiting room, totally broken. It was tough to be left there alone (among) all the others, with my wet red eyes. It (would have) been better to sit in another room and not be exposed to all the others. After these examinations, I had to wait for the test results for several days; this was a new, terrible period. The doctor would call me as soon (as) he had the answer, but I was certain of having cancer. I decided to tell my husband before the doctor gave me the final answer. He (was) more shocked than me; I felt (that) I was inflicting pain on him and that it was my fault.

After approximately a week, the doctor called me while I was sitting in my car on my way to work. I stopped the car to hear his message. Finally, it was confirmed; I had cancer. The diagnosis felt unreal. The world changed quickly and dramatically. I felt physically well but had just learned that I had a serious disease. In a way, I felt healthy but had to adapt to a serious diagnosis. I felt well and sick at the same time. It (was) just amazing how different everything (had) been since I got the diagnosis. To avoid (being) overwhelmed by (my) feelings, I had to distance (myself) emotionally from the reality. I said to myself, 'This message is not about me'. If

I (would) manage to do my job, I had to 'push away' (these thoughts) and find something else to think about. I tried to push the thoughts away, but somehow, the thoughts always returned. I kept the mask, but I was in an emotional chaos. Different emotions came in waves. Several times, I had to rush to the toilet, and several times, I broke out in a cold sweat.

Curative treatment phase

Then I had to wait for surgery. It was so frantic – all that happened the first months – that I (had) trouble remembering everything, but I (did) not care to remember it either because it was a terrible time. Every morning, I woke up (with the) thought (that) I (had) cancer. It was a terrible, hopeless feeling. It created a great vacuum for me; I was in a catastrophe and terribly scared. It was difficult to receive the information I needed. In spite of being informed that I could call health professionals when needed, I was afraid of disturbing them. In addition, it (was) not easy to call somebody (whom I had) never met before.

When I got (the) date of (the) surgery, it alleviated my fear and anxiety and gave me a sense of security and control; finally, something was happening. It (was) easier to relate to something concrete even if the treatment could be very hard. I didn't mind losing my breast. I (didn't) connect (my) identity and feelings to it. If the doctors had told me that my prognosis would be better by (their) taking (out) both breasts, they could! What was of importance for me all this time was to get rid of the cancer; the loss of a breast was of minor importance.

After surgery, I had some terrible experiences. When I went (for) chemo, I was so low in white blood cells that I was (placed in) solitary confinement twice. It was such a horrendous experience; I thought that this (was) how it (felt) to sit in jail. (I was) in the room, and (I) look(ed) at the closed door, and (I) hear(d) the sounds outside, and (I was) completely left to (myself). I had never thought that within 48 hours, I would be a nervous wreck. I like(d) to have control of the time schedule of my treatment, but the nurses forgot, and they (were) too busy. Health professionals are in a hurry; you can see it right away by the look in their eyes. Sometimes, I did not bother to connect with them because I knew they had to 'run' before (I) finished the sentence. It's gotten worse and worse, more and more patients, not more employees; they are 'running' all day when they are at work. (It) does not feel good for them, and it does not feel good for us.

It was terrible to lose my hair; now everyone could see that I was sick. Suddenly, I looked completely different. I isolated myself from others. (W)hen I got the wig, I still felt different. Those who did not know my story could ask, 'What have you done with your hair'?

(There was a) very big difference in how people (related to me); sometimes, I felt that I was treated as a diagnosis and a number in the row, while others managed to see me as a person.

Palliative phase

One day, the doctor told me (that) there were no more treatment options left to offer and that it was doubtful that I (would) experience (the next) Christmas. There and then, it was half a year (before) Christmas. Now I felt sicker than ever, but I would no longer be a patient at the cancer ward although it was at the cancer ward (where) I was most familiar. To receive (the) message that the disease (was) incurable and that they (had) no more treatment to offer (was) hard, but it (was) also very difficult that I (did) not know (to) which hospital ward I belong(ed). I (had) completed the curative treatment at the cancer ward, but I (was) still in need of their professional care, and in the cancer ward, they (knew) me. Now, everyone (would be) discharged from (the) hospital regardless of how sick (one was). I had to return home despite my weakness and pain, without knowing where to go if my situation suddenly (got) worse, and I need(ed) instant help. My husband and children (could not) be with me all the time. But I need(ed) help; I need(ed) people around me who (could) help me when I need(ed) it. I (felt) unsafe. Now they must find a place for me where I (could stay).

In my situation, it (was) challenging to ask for help, especially when the different nurses who (came) and (went were) so busy. It (was) like I (was) squeezing their already busy time schedule. My cancer (had) spread to (my) lungs, and it (was) hard to breathe; when I (was) dependent on oxygen and drugs, I (felt) unsafe at home. Home nurses (came), but they (left) again, and it (would) always take some time before they (would return). They (were) not there at the moment (when) I need(ed) them. What I (wanted at that) time (was) to be safe and to have confidence that the healthcare system (would) take care of this last part of my life. Confidence (was) what it (would) be about in the days to come. In (that) situation, I wish(ed) that I was offered help instead of having to ask for help. For then, I (would have) received time instead of (having) to take others' time. If you care(d), you (would) do your priorities by your heart, not by your head. (The fact) that some (came) to (me) when (I was) hot and sweaty and (they) turn(ed) the pillow without (my) having to ask for it mean(t) so much. It (was) such a small thing to do, but it (was) great to get a cool pad (on) the neck. Some (would) see it; others (would) not see it.

Now I am very grateful to have been admitted to the palliative care ward although I do not know how long I will be here. I will at least be here (until) next week. When I (first) came in here, everything was hopeless; the pain overwhelmed me, and I did not want to live anymore. Here it is absolutely fantastic; now I feel a new desire to live in the time I have left. One day, I was crying in bed; a nurse came in and just sat there until I had no more tears. It was of great importance. Elsewhere, they look at the clock all the time and are not present; they come in with painkillers and a glass of water and say, 'drink this' and leave again.

Critical thinking activities

1 What are the characteristic signs that show when the caring part is either evident or absent in care? Write a paragraph reflecting on the most important aspects of caring.

2 What was the most important lesson for you after reading this narrative?

3 Read through the narrative once more, with this question in mind: which notion of dignity is most prominent in Mary's story?

Discussion

In our view, the four notions of dignity are present in relation, action and morality and are therefore related in different ways to Martinsen's (2006) theory of care. Care has become something it is not, such as a public service in which both relation and morality may be missing. Dignity is a core aspect in both care and caring. Dignity consists of inherent and external dimensions, which are common to all humans and, at the same time, unique to each individual. On the basis of Mary's story, we now discuss how the four notions of dignity are present in the three dimensions of care.

Based on our experiences and research, the four notions of dignity are all essential in the context of illness and the subject's self-image. This issue becomes apparent in the way we are being cared for and treated.

As stated earlier, the first notion of dignity is called *the universal human dignity (Menschenwürde)*. This kind of dignity does not vary but is associated with being human and basic human rights – everyone has the right to be treated with the same degree of respect. However, what varies is how health professionals safeguard universal human dignity in terms of relation, action and morality. The last three notions of dignity depend on relationships, circumstances and contexts, which may vary, as illustrated below.

Human dignity is safeguarded (or not) by the way people act morally or otherwise in their relationships with others. We will now interpret and discuss the concept of dignity in relation to Martinsen's philosophy of caring, which consists of three dimensions – relation, action and morality (Alvsvåg 2010, p. 173; Martinsen 2003, pp. 15–16). However, both care and dignity are ambiguous concepts (Alvsvåg 2010; Martinsen 2003; Nordenfelt 2004; Nordenfelt & Edgar 2005). When people are afflicted by serious diseases, their dependence on others becomes evident. At such times, they need more than simply to receive care. *How* care is applied is at the heart of the concept of caring. Furthermore, the four notions of dignity are overlapping and interconnected, despite their differences. In specific human relationships, some of the notions of dignity can be more visible than others.

Relation

Caring has been described as a human trait, a moral imperative, an interpersonal relationship and a therapeutic intervention and affect (Morse *et al.* 2000). The moral stature of individuals is reflected in their relations. The actions of the individuals in a relationship have an impact on preserving their dignity of identity (Nordenfelt 2004). In the context of illness, this means being regarded as human, rather than 'a diagnosis being treated' (Drageset *et al.* 2015).

Martinsen (2006) distinguishes between 'a registering eye' and 'the eye of the heart' – in other words, being perceived as a diagnosis versus being seen as an individual. When someone sees with 'the recording eye', they withdraw from the situation, and no real interaction takes place in the room. 'The eye puts itself in an outside position, busy with looking for and abstracting common characteristics to organise these under an already defined concept or classification' (Martinsen 2006, p. 97). When we 'register' something, we are concerned with what is the same, such as typical physical signs and symptoms. In contrast, 'Seeing with the heart's eye, with the participating, attentive eye, makes the other emerge as significant' (Martinsen 2006, p. 86). Professional knowledge about the patient includes seeing the person behind the disease, as a unique individual. We need to remember that there is a unique human being behind every diagnosis, with a distinct life story. If we do not view another human being as a unique person, we are in danger of violating their dignity of identity.

In our story, Mary wants to be seen, understood and respected as an individual. Despite her needs, she sometimes feels she is being treated as a diagnosis. In this situation and according to Nordenfelt and Edgar (2005), Mary's dignity is either protected or violated, and she perceives the care provided as either caring or careless. Nurses should never take for granted that they fully understand their patients (Ellingsen *et al.* 2015). It is the person receiving the care who determines whether it is caring or careless. This person also decides whether their dignity is protected or violated. Mary's dignity is protected when the doctor takes her seriously at once and listens to her. On the contrary, she feels violated when she is left feeling totally broken and alone among other unknown patients, exposed to them with her wet red eyes. Such a relationship (where caring is lacking in care) may threaten a person's self-respect and integrity.

Another example can illustrate the violation of dignity. For Mary, the loss of her breast has less significance; her major concern is the loss of her hair. This case demonstrates that the gaze of others can potentially violate a person's dignity. Losing one's hair is visible to others. In this situation, the gaze of others is interpreted as threatening Mary's self-esteem and thereby her dignity. Dignity is relational, as it includes both how the individual is seen and treated by others.

Action

The moral stature of the individual is directly dependent on the person's attitude, which is reflected in action, as depicted in this narrative about the relationship between the health professionals and the patient (Nordenfelt 2004). In other words, the health professionals' attitudes have effects on how the patient's dignity is safeguarded. According to Martinsen, without action, caring is reduced to sentimental emotions (Alvsvåg 2010, p. 173). What the action in care comprises and how it should be performed is situationally, professionally and culturally dependent but always justified by the individual in need of care. This issue is exemplified in the episode when Mary is lying in bed, hot and sweaty; without her having to ask for help, the nurse comes in, turns the pillow and gives her a cool pad for her neck. It is the caring part in care that makes a vital difference in protecting the individual's dignity. The awareness of such dignity when performing nursing activities prevents care from becoming inhuman and technological. 'The ignorant eyes of the busy world see the worth of humans only as related to activity and productivity. The heart's eye, the participating, attentive eye, sees the significant in all human life and lets it exist as itself' (Martinsen 2006, p. 95). This is what it means to see with the heart's eye and thus protect the individual's dignity. The person who masters seeing with the heart's eye is naturally invited to attend to the patient's condition to find out what serves them best. This places the nurse in a participating position where the patient is a significant person (Martinsen 2006, p. 97). Caring means the way or manner in which care is performed, and this is exemplified when Mary is crying in bed, and the nurse sees her need and is present in Mary's suffering.

Morality

The attributes of preserving dignity are individualised care, restored control, respect, advocacy and sensitive listening. The antecedents are professional knowledge, responsibility, reflection and non-hierarchical organisation. The consequences are strengthening the life spirit, an inner sense of freedom, self-respect and successful coping (Anderberg *et al.* 2007). Treatment and care can be executed by following evidence-based guidelines, but the patient may still feel offended by the way this care or treatment is performed. Morality is therefore the third dimension of care and refers to our way of being in the relationship and the manner in which the action is performed. Morality is demonstrated in how the individual is viewed and treated, which is connected to dignity and also to caring in care.

Respect comes from the Latin word *re-spectare*, meaning 'look again'; we need to look again and see the person behind the diagnosis. Respect is related to morality in many ways (Nordenfelt 2004). According to Nordenfelt and Edgar (2005), protecting the dignity of moral stature and identity implies that the care is individualised to perform the deeds of value to the individual, where the subject's self-respect and integrity of body and mind are preserved. However, what this matter constitutes may vary from situation to situation and from patient to patient. This aspect is also illustrated in Finfgeld-Connett's (2008) meta-synthesis, describing that caring in nursing is a context-specific interpersonal process characterised by expert nursing practice, interpersonal sensitivity and intimate relationships. This view may be challenged in a healthcare system that emphasises rapidity and registration, which may lead to an attitude that is not marked with sensitivity but deadlock (Martinsen, 2006, p. 61). This issue is exemplified in the story of Mary, when she feels treated like a diagnosis and not as a person.

Despite the ideal of independence, as human beings, we are always dependent on others. When we are newborn, this is evident. However, this fact can be easily forgotten in a normal, healthy life. Today, dependence on others can be considered a weakness (Toombs 2004). We live in relationships with and reliant on one another, but when a person is forced into a vulnerable situation, this dependency becomes more evident. In healthcare, the professionals are in a position of power in relation to their patients. The healthcare professionals must be aware of this imbalance and exercise their power by means of caring judgement. However, one of the most powerful barriers to retaining a sense of dignity in illness is the prevailing cultural perspective on autonomy that prominently features the attributes and values of self-reliance, involving the capacity to provide for one's own needs without another's help (Toombs 2004). The fact that we are all dependent on one another appears to contradict the notion of autonomy. Maybe this is why Mary has to ask for help instead of being offered it. We believe that this is a misunderstanding of the concept. Autonomy is about preserving the person's dignity. It is the way care is performed – the caring part in care – that takes care of the individual's dignity. When Mary is offered help, she feels that she has received time; in this way, her humanity is affirmed. In contrast, when she has to ask for help, her vulnerability and helplessness are confirmed (Ellingsen *et al.* 2013).

Chapter summary

- In the story of Mary, dignity is illuminated as the caring part in care. Dignity and care are connected. The caring part in care is evident in how the patient is being seen, heard, understood and treated as a person. Dignity is safeguarded by the caring part in care.

- If caring is absent in care, patients may feel that their dignity is being violated. Violated dignity might lead to increased suffering.

- Reflection is crucial for the nurse to preserve human dignity in care.

- Caring is an act that takes care of life, with consideration for the other person. To preserve dignity in care, it is necessary to be aware of the patient's individual needs for care, respect, advocacy and sensitive listening.

Suggested reading

For more in-depth understanding, you are encouraged to read:

Alvsvåg, H. (2010). 'Kari Martinsen: Philosophy of Caring' in A. Marriner-Tomey & M.R. Alligood (eds) *Nursing theorists and their work*. St Louis, MO: Mosby Elsevier. pp. 165–187.

Martinsen, K. (2006). *Care and vulnerability*. Oslo: Akribe.

Nordenfelt, L. (2004). The varieties of dignity. *Health Care Analysis: Journal of Health Philosophy and Policy*. **12**, 69–81.

Nordenfelt, L. & Edgar, A. (2005). The four notions of dignity. *Quality in Ageing*. **6**(1), 17–21.

References

Alvsvåg, H. (2010). 'Kari Martinsen: Philosophy of Caring' in A. Marriner-Tomey & M.R. Alligood (eds) *Nursing theorists and their work*. St Louis, MO: Mosby Elsevier. pp. 165–187.

Anderberg, P., Lepp, M., Berglund, A-L. & Segesten, K. (2007). Preserving dignity in caring for older adults: a concept analysis. *Journal of Advanced Nursing*. **59**(6), 635–43.

Drageset, S., Lindstrøm, T.C. & Underlid, K. (2010). Coping with breast cancer: between diagnosis and surgery. *Journal of Advanced Nursing*. **66**, 149–58.

Drageset, S., Lindstrøm, T.C., Giske, T. & Underlid, K. (2011). Being in suspense: women's experiences awaiting breast cancer surgery. *Journal of Advanced Nursing*. **67**, 1941–51.

Drageset, S., Lindstrøm, T.C., Giske, T. & Underlid, K. (2012). 'The support I need': Women's experiences of social support after having received breast cancer diagnosis and awaiting surgery. *Cancer Nursing*. **35**, 39–47.

Drageset, S., Lindstrøm, T. C., Giske, T. & Underlid, K. (2015). Women's experiences of social support during the first year following primary breast cancer surgery. *Scandinavian Journal of Caring Sciences*.10.1111/scs.12250.

Ellingsen, Sidsel (2015). *Tiden i livet og livet i tiden. Opplevelse av tid ved langkommet uhelbredelig sykdom. [Time in life and life in time. Experiences of time when living with incurable disease]* PhD Thesis, University in Bergen, Norway.

Ellingsen, Sidsel, Roxberg, Åsa, Kristoffersen, Kjell, Rosland, Jan Henrik & Alvsvåg, Herdis (2013). To enter a world with no future A phenomenological study describing the embodied experience of time when living with severe incurable disease. *Scandinavian Journal of Caring Sciences*, **27** (1): 165–74. doi:10.1111/j.1471-6712.201201019.

Ellingsen, Sidsel, Roxberg, Åsa, Kristoffersen, Kjell, Rosland, Jan Henrik & Alvsvåg Herdis (2014). Being in transit and in transition. The experience of time at the place, when living with severe incurable disease – a phenomenological study. *Scandinavian Journal of Caring Sciences*. **28** (3), 458–68. doi: 10.1111/scs.12067.

Ellingsen, Sidsel, Roxberg, Åsa, Kristoffersen, Kjell, Rosland, Jan Henrik & Alvsvåg Herdis (2015). The pendulum time of life. The experience of time, when living with severe incurable disease: Phenomenological and philosophical study. *Medicine, Healthcare and Philosophy*. **18**(2), 203–15. doi: 10.1007/s11019-014-9590-9

Finfgeld-Connett, D. (2008). Meta-synthesis of caring in nursing. *Journal of Clinical Nursing*. **17**, 196–204.

Global Dignity Norway (2015). http://www.globaldignity.no/ (accessed 26 May 2016).

Martinsen, Kari (2003). *Omsorg, sykepleie, medisin*. 2nd edn. Norway: Universitetsforlaget.

Martinsen, Kari (2006). *Care and vulnerability*. Oslo, Norway: Akribe.

Morse, J. (2000). Responding to the cues of suffering. *Health Care Women International*. **21**(1), 1–9.

Nordenfelt, L. (2004). The varieties of dignity. *Health care analysis: HCA: journal of health philosophy and policy*. **12**, 69–81.

Nordenfelt, L. & Edgar, A. (2005). The four notions of dignity. *Quality in Ageing*. **6**(1), 17–21

Toombs, S. Kay (2004). Living and dying with dignity: Reflections on lived experience. *Journal of Palliative Care*. **20**(3), 193–200.

World Health Organization (2015). *Globocan 2012: Estimated Cancer Incidence, Mortality and Prevalence Worldwide in 2012*. http://globocan.iarc.fr/Pages/fact_sheets_population.aspx (accessed 26 May 2016).

Chapter 5

Storytelling as a dignity-preserving practice in palliative care

Oddgeir Synnes

Introduction

For American literary critic Anatole Broyard, a prostate cancer diagnosis produced a creative spark of writings about his illness. In his memoir *Intoxicated by my illness*, published after his death, Broyard states, 'It may not be dying we fear so much, but the diminished self' (1992, p. 25). Broyard's fear of a diminished self makes for compelling reading, as he argues that patients need to start treating their illnesses as an occasion for stories.

I have been using storytelling for several years in my work with patients in palliative care. In this chapter, I will argue that stories can provide some sort of stability in the face of an uncertain and threatening future. This is largely because stories are not mere representations of reality but actually constitute the way we look at ourselves. Experiences are not given; they are discovered through language. In this way, language and stories are linked to identity. Anthony Giddens stresses this, with his argument that a person's identity is found 'in the capacity *to keep a particular narrative going*' (1991, p. 54).

I will put forward an understanding of storytelling as an attempt to keep a particular narrative going in the face of death, using examples from my own work with storytelling among dying cancer patients. This storytelling practice must be seen as closely related to dignity, as in Nordenfelt and Edgar's (2005) theory, which argues that the dignity of identity might be lost when one encounters a serious illness. By tying narrative, identity and dignity together, I will argue that a storytelling practice can be one way of confronting the fear of a 'diminished self'.

Learning objectives

This chapter will enable you to:

- Understand how stories of illness are closely related to identity and dignity
- Reflect on how dignity can be maintained through the act of storytelling
- Get an insight into the complex meaning construction that is at stake in the stories of patients suffering from a terminal illness

Dignity of identity and illness

In their article 'The four notions of dignity', Nordenfelt and Edgar (2005) propose four different understandings of dignity in an attempt to clarify the various implications for understanding dignity in care for older people: (1) dignity of merit; (2) dignity of moral stature; (3) dignity of identity; and (4) universal dignity or *Menschenwürde*. According to Nordenfelt and Edgar (2005), dignity of identity (which relates to a person's integrity and identity as a human being) is the hardest to define. Yet they see it as the most important aspect of dignity in relation to illness and old age because 'this kind of dignity can be taken from us by external events, such as the acts of other people, as well as by injury, illness and old age […] It is the dignity that we attach to ourselves as integrated and autonomous persons, persons with a history and persons with a future' (Nordenfelt & Edgar 2005, p. 19).

Examples of events that might compromise our sense of dignity of identity are bodily damage, irreversible disablement, the violation of integrity by carers upon whom we are dependent, social exclusion and so forth. An important aspect of the dignity of identity is that there are events or actions that put our understanding of who we are under threat. Indeed, beyond this threat, we might even lose our self-understanding and self-respect (Nordenfelt 2004). Therefore, it is this understanding of dignity – dignity of identity – that I would like to emphasise in a narrative understanding in healthcare. As the above quotation shows, the dignity of identity is vulnerable to illness. Furthermore, this dignity is related to a sense of continuity by having a history and possessing a hope for the future, which a serious illness might threaten. Though Nordenfelt and Edgar (2005) do not relate this to a narrative understanding, it seems clear that the notion of dignity of identity would encompass a narrative understanding.

Narrative identity and the need for stories in illness

Identity is a contested topic. However, the increasing emphasis on narrative in the humanities and social sciences, as well as in medicine and healthcare, has led to a growing interest in, and understanding of, personal identity in the context of a narrative. According to this view, identity is not a core or a substance of the inner self but a result of what happens in one's life and how one responds to this through interpretation (Ritivoi 2008). Several theorists have argued that narrative and identity are tied together through the provision of continuity to the self (Giddens 1991, MacIntyre 2007, Ricoeur 1992, Taylor 1989).

According to the French philosopher Paul Ricoeur (1988), stories articulate time and make time 'human' by integrating the past, present and future. We tell a story by interpreting the past in the light of the present, and thus prepare for the future. But, in some instances, this can require considerable effort. Here, we can see a relationship between a narrative understanding and Nordenfelt and Edgar's (2005) understanding of dignity of identity as something that requires a history. In other words, the loss of a story equals the loss of personal identity, which in turn equals loss of the dignity of identity. Thus, narrative identity is vulnerable to various experiences and occurrences that might require a new understanding or a new plot to fit with unexpected events. In some instances, therefore, we can talk of a loss of narrative identity (Ricoeur 1992). As philosopher Alasdair MacIntyre argues, 'When someone complains [...] that his or her life is meaningless, he or she is often and perhaps characteristically complaining that the narrative of their life has become unintelligible to them, that it lacks any point, any movement towards a climax or a *telos*' (2007, p. 217).

As shown above, narrative identity is closely connected to meaning-making when one experiences various significant events throughout one's life. Therefore, it is not surprising that this notion of narrative has become influential in understanding illness (Charon 2006, Frank 1995, Mattingly 1998). In this tradition of 'illness narratives', serious illness is seen not just as a biological breakdown but equally as a biographical one (Bury 1982), which can imply a loss of self (Charmaz 1983) that must be met with a narrative reconstruction (Williams 1984). As Arthur W. Frank, one of the leading voices in the literature on illness narratives, puts it, 'Becoming seriously ill is a call for stories [...] Stories have to repair the damage that illness has done to the ill person's sense of where she is in life, and where she may be going. Stories are a way of redrawing maps and finding new destinations' (1995, p. 53).

The focus of this chapter

In this chapter, I will advocate the adoption of a storytelling practice in palliative care that is based on the previous remarks concerning dignity of identity and narrative identity. I will propose an argument for storytelling as a way of preserving or upholding a narrative identity, which I regard as a vital aspect of upholding the dignity of identity. I will do this by taking a detour through the stories of particular palliative care patients. What I would like to do is show how storytelling can be seen as a way of upholding or recreating oneself through narrative. But I will also demonstrate why this can be difficult to achieve in some stories. The chapter will conclude with a discussion of *narrative care*, emphasising the need not just for stories but for the mutual relationship that exists between storytellers and listeners.

Storytelling among palliative care patients

Terminally ill patients are among the most vulnerable patients in healthcare settings. Cicely Saunders (1996, 2001), the founder of modern hospice care and philosophy, argued for the importance of implementing storytelling in palliative care. Though palliative care still adopts a predominantly biomedical and symptom-relieving approach (Ragan *et al.* 2003), there is an increasing focus on patients' existential and spiritual needs and challenges. Although the role of narrative in palliative care is expanding, it is still in its infancy (Thomas *et al.* 2009, p. 788), and the research is diverse and fragmented (Gunaratnam & Oliviere 2009).

In 2006–2007, I was leading a project concerning the existential needs of palliative care patients. During this period, I taught six courses in writing and storytelling; three were held at a palliative care unit in a nursing home and three were conducted in a day-care setting at a palliative care clinic. The work resulted in roughly 300 pages and about 450 stories from 51 participants between the ages of 43 and 94 years. The project was founded on the belief that storytelling could make a valuable contribution to a holistic approach in the existential care of palliative care patients. Hence, it was not an academic research project, although I used the stories later as the prime empirical material in my PhD thesis (Synnes 2012). In the following sections, I will describe and demonstrate how an understanding of the practical experiences from the storytelling courses, in conjunction with some of the main findings in my thesis, may offer a fruitful way of maintaining the dignity of identity.

Contrary to most research on illness narratives, I was not primarily interested in what the participants had to say about their illness and their interpretation of it. Rather, I wanted the participants to write or discuss what they wanted to talk about. Therefore, I gave them specific, open-ended exercises or narrative prompts, which allowed them to decide what they wanted to talk about. These narrative prompts included phrases such as 'that day', 'I never told anybody', 'if I could go back to one place', 'everyday life', 'the meeting' and 'the future'. I never specifically asked the participants about their disease, but for many of them, this became an important aspect – though never the sole focus. Others did not want to discuss their illness but wanted to focus instead on other aspects of their lives.

Despite the heterogeneity of the stories, they share some common features. What is at stake in the stories, and in the practice of storytelling, is a striving to uphold oneself, sometimes through a reconfiguration of oneself. But this is a fragile enterprise and, in certain situations, the narrative self is lost. Of course, stories are a construction and do not present the whole truth of a patient's inner world. Nevertheless, they are the self's medium of being (Frank 2010) and, as such, offer valuable insights into a patient's perception of the here and now, their past life and their vision for the future. When Nordenfelt and Edgar (2005) suggest that human dignity is related to the experience of continued personal history, with a vision for the future, this can be applied to a narrative understanding and practice. In this chapter, I aim to show how a narrative identity can be understood as a means of preserving the human dignity in palliative patients' stories about illness as well as other aspects of their lives.

Stories of illness as dignity of identity

My participants' stories of illness can be regarded as stories that strive for the continuity of narrative identity. The challenge is how to interpret a life-threatening disease as part of one's ongoing story. In some cases, the narrator manages to turn the disease into a continuation of their previous life. The illness becomes manageable by interpreting the present in the light of the past, as in this account from an 80-year-old woman in a palliative care unit, at a nursing home:

> I have experienced a lot of illness throughout my life (...) When I look back, I think that after all, I have had a good life. Jesus makes my life lighter. He helps me now too. I am not afraid to die. The doctors were so astonished at my reaction when I was diagnosed and got to know that I probably would die in a short time, that I could be so cold and quiet. Cold and quiet? I reacted with strong emotions!
>
> I've been lying in bed screaming today. I have had terrible pains. Nausea, I've always found, has been worse than pain, but these pains are the worst. I cannot bear the thought of food.
>
> No, I do not think these are long days. But I would not have managed without Jesus. He has been with me all my life. As a child, my father took me to the children's worship in the church.
>
> And I have been a Sunday school teacher for many years...

This is an excerpt from a longer story that mentions various losses throughout the woman's life. She has experienced the support and strength of Jesus when encountering loss and illness, and these experiences have given her the strength to deal with the present situation and come to terms with it. Thus, the present and even the future become bearable, despite the intolerable pain that she is enduring ('I am not afraid to die'). What we are presented with is a narrative understanding; without her history, and the support that she gains from it, neither we nor she could understand the outcome of the story as anything other than a claim.

At other times, however, the narrator does not find support in the past, and instead of calling on resources from the past, must find resources in the present, as in the following story from a 53-year-old woman at a day-care unit:

The day ... I discovered that I was happy, I had been told that I was seriously ill, that I might not live much longer.

But I was not sad, though I often cried and sometimes at inappropriate occasions. But, at the same time, I carried an overwhelming feeling of happiness.

I got many visits at the hospital. Many were upset that I was sick. People collected money for me to go to a hospital abroad and get alternative treatment. The doctors, nurses and others in healthcare were caring.

And I got so much more than I had the sense to ask for. I got letters and cards; friends called and asked if they could do anything for me. I learned that friends had made a list for when to call me, so they would not bother me too much; friends redecorated my bedroom. I got an offer to go on tours, travel domestically and overseas; my children said that I was irreplaceable.

So, I was not sad; I was happy.

Here, the narrator is not establishing the continuity of her narrative identity. Instead, she needs to accommodate a new perspective on herself and her illness. The illness becomes a change that establishes a new direction – a new continuity that links the present to a possible future involving hope. But how does this relate to human dignity? It is tied to the understanding that stories are not just mirrors of our inner selves but are a medium through which we can articulate and find meaning. As Paul Ricoeur stresses, 'The inscription of discourse is the transcription of the world, and transcription is not reduplication, but metamorphosis' (1976, p. 42). By giving patients the opportunity to share their stories of their experiences of illness, we also enable them to provide coherence and find new directions in their illness. Stories are a way of putting oneself in a perspective that is bearable. As Ricoeur argues in a later work, 'The plot "redeems" the origin of the "fall" into meaninglessness' (1992, p. 142). Experiences are not given; they are created. Through creative imagination, and by putting our confused and chaotic situation into a plot that makes sense, we can make the unbearable endurable.

However, this is not always the case. Tragedy can sometimes be too devastating for us to accommodate in a meaningful plot. We may experience a loss of coherence and continuity – what Arthur W. Frank (1995) calls 'a chaos narrative'. One example of this is the following story of a male participant, aged 54, attending a day-care unit:

What is everyday life today? There is something missing; something that I cannot find; something unworried that has gone into hiding...

When I go on a diet, I have almost no symptoms of the cancer. It's a little bit strange, but it's also good because, then, the cancer can nearly be forgotten.

It's almost like the everyday life I had before I got sick. But that's definitely not true. So, how is it, then? (…) Where has the everyday life disappeared? This is scary. I have not really thought about this before – what exactly is my everyday life now?

Before I got ill, everyday life was the dull, boring days that always repeated themselves, the days that I tried to avoid to have a meaningful life. Now, it seems that it's the old everyday life I long for, but that is an impossible wish, since it has disappeared. My days now consist of waiting – waiting for results, waiting for treatment, waiting to get sick of treatment and waiting to get good from treatment. But it can't be waiting that is my everyday life now; that is too depressing. So, where in the world has my everyday life gone? (...)

Now, I have decided to put the thoughts of my everyday life aside. Maybe some good thoughts will appear. Nothing much happens these days. It's like life itself has slowed down in its own quiet rhythm. But time goes fast. Very fast. Tuesdays are like beads on a string. It's almost like I'm thinking, 'I was at the day ward the other day. I don't think I'll bother going today.'

Can it really be this that has become my everyday life now? Days that disappear so fast? Days that disappear almost without content and without me noticing that they are gone? Then that will mean that my last days alive will disappear too without me even noticing. Then, what's the point...

In the story above, there is no direction, no way out of the chaos or despair, for the narrator. Everyday life has collapsed into a meaningless existence, where there is no link between the present and the past. The everyday life that was previously characterised by an unworried existence has been replaced by an everyday life of uncertainty and depressive thoughts. And the knowledge that this newfound everyday life will, in the not too distant future, lead to the narrator's death makes it impossible to offer a positive interpretation of the present. Thus, the narrative ends without a clear purpose: 'Then, what's the point...'

Frank (1995) argues that real chaos narratives cannot be told. A certain degree of telling or configuration implies some sort of order, a processing through language. I will argue that this story is not truly about chaos; rather, it is a story of *despair*. Consequently, it is a story that shows the lack of continuity of a narrative identity or a case of the narrative identity being under threat. However, I will also argue that this kind of story is an example of how storytelling can be seen as an important aspect of preserving a patient's dignity. The telling of stories, whether they are chaotic or stories of despair, represents a 'therapeutic opening' (Frank 1998, p. 202).

As the above narrator says, he could not talk about his everyday life – because it had disappeared. But when we met the next time, he had written this particular story. The story became a way of narrating an experience that he had been unable to put into words, by making the unsayable narratable. The story therefore came to represent an affirmation of the narrator's experiences that had previously been mute and unarticulated. And the sharing of this story with other patients represented another level of affirmation. The listeners gave the storyteller an *audience* that acknowledged the telling. Another important aspect was how the story came to serve as a *connector* between the narrator and the other patients. After reading this narrative, several of the participants responded to the story and to the narrator by saying that this story had articulated many of their own experiences, and that this resulted in a common understanding that they were both able to acknowledge and share in further discussions.

Upholding the dignity of identity through stories where illness is absent

Stories of illness are only one part of the multi-faceted body of stories that my participants shared. Though the stories of illness were obviously a very important issue for many of the storytellers; for others, this was only one aspect among many, and some barely mentioned illness. The stories were all told in the context of palliative care, but it would be a misjudgement to assume that everyone who is ill is predominantly occupied with illness. As Norwegian anthropologist Unni Wikan (2000) argues, the stories of ill people may not just be stories about illness; if we are only asking about the illness, we may leave out what is of the greatest concern to the ill. Although Wikan is speaking from the perspective of the researcher, this is a crucial point for healthcare professionals to remember as well. Research involving seriously ill cancer patients has shown that not all patients want to discuss their illness or worries; though they would like to be given the opportunity to do so by healthcare staff, ultimately, they wish to decide for themselves (Edwards 2005, Kvåle 2007, Thulesius *et al.* 2003). However, this research also stresses the need for patients to be able to share other aspects of their lives as part of an existential care requiring an interested listener. This is also a central point in the understanding of spiritual care in palliative care, where listening to the patient in light of their life story is seen as vital (Murray 2002, Nolan 2011, Saunders 2003).

In my encounters with the storytellers and their stories, I soon realised that it required an openness from me to what the patients themselves wanted to talk about. At one of the meetings at the day-care unit, I gave the narrative prompt 'This has been important in your life'. The youngest participant, a 43-year-old woman, responded with the following poem:

> You're asking me about what
> has been important in my life
> as it is already in the past
>
> but don't you realise
>
> my life was threatened
> before I had learned to love it
>
> my life was destroyed
> before I had dared to live it
>
> don't ask me about what
> has been
> ask me about what
> is

The woman was clearly provoked by this particular exercise. She did not want to talk about what *had been* the important part of her life, as it was already over. (I must admit that it was an ill-informed choice of exercise!) Instead, she wanted to talk about her life here and now, her thoughts about her experience with the illness, but not least about her everyday life that she could still enjoy without it being totally disrupted by her illness. The woman's rebellion against my narrative prompt constitutes a *performative act of dignity.* By writing a poem, she preserves her dignity by refusing to let her life exist in the past. In the poem, she demands that we ask about what is still there in her life.

Many of the participants' stories can be seen as their own answers to this very question. These are stories that predominantly stress the possibility of continuity between their life before illness and their everyday life now. Examples of this are stories about continuing participation in family life, of still being able to do everyday tasks, and so on. But even though these stories represent a form of continuity with their previous lives, their importance lies precisely in their newfound value and the fact that this sense of continuity is fragile and is no longer something that can be taken for granted. An example of this is the woman who triumphantly declared her decision to buy a new car. She refused to let the fact that she might not be able to drive it for very long hinder her joy and sense of expectation.

On the other hand, upholding the continuity of one's everyday life is not easy, and many of the participants, especially those in the inpatient unit, had almost lost hope of being able to preserve some sort of permanence in their present situation. An 80-year-old gentleman in the inpatient unit gave the following response when asked about his day that day:

> I am not thinking much about the day today
> I am thinking about earlier stuff
> About my childhood, my family
> About all kinds of things
> But not the day today

Here, we see a totally opposite attitude to that in the poem written by the 43-year-old woman. Whereas *she* refuses to contemplate the past, others can find meaning and a confirmation of their previous life by talking about it.

Stories of the past can be divided into two categories. The first category consists of stories of significant positive and negative events throughout life that provide new direction and show development in the narrator's life story. The telling of such stories can be considered in relation to the term 'integrative reminiscence' (Rybarczyk & Bellg 1997), where significant events are told and integrated into the continuing story of who one is. These are stories that show a particular development or new direction in the narrator's life story. These kinds of stories therefore offer an insight into how the storyteller has become who they are today.

The second category comprises stories about lighter memories from childhood and youth. In contrast to most research on narrative and identity, these stories are not about change. On the contrary, they are characterised by the fact that nothing in particular happens. They are idyllic and nostalgic glimpses of a previous life that was simpler. But it would be a fallacy to dismiss these lighter stories of the past as escapism. In his book *Yearning for yesterday: a sociology of nostalgia* (1979), Fred Davis argues that the primary purpose of nostalgia is to facilitate the continuity of identity. Routledge *et al.* (2011) find that a threat to existential meaning can act as a trigger for nostalgia, and Deciou Ritivoi (2002) considers nostalgia as a safety net that can give a sense of grounding and stability. I read these stories of nostalgia as a way of upholding a sense of continuity in a situation of total discontinuity, by focusing on positive memories in a difficult everyday life, where death is imminent (Synnes 2015).

The lighter stories of the past are also enjoyable, easily tellable, do not require much of the storyteller and involve little risk. At the same time, they offer valuable identity signifiers through the appearance of central characters and a particular environment, as we hear about parents, grandparents, siblings and friends, all in the specific setting of their childhood home, the streets of their home town and so forth. This illustrates Ricoeur's (1992) argument that a narrative understanding refuses to let us see people as isolated, because stories require other people. Even in the small, seemingly insignificant lighter stories of the past, the narrator emerges with a particularity among significant others in a distinctive environment.

The stories of the past are another version of *rising to the occasion* (May 1991, quoted in Frank 1995, p. 62) that illness represents. The stories can be seen as a way of maintaining a part of the narrator's identity that is not totally dominated by illness. The narrator in this case may be a dying elderly woman, but she still has her memories, and through the act of storytelling she can give glimpses of who she once was and what are still parts of her. As Frank argues, 'Dying is not a loss of the old map and destination…' (1995, p. 162).

Critical thinking activities

1. What is the common denominator of dignity in the stories of the palliative patients that you read above?
2. How do these stories correspond to stories you have encountered in your own practice as a student or as a healthcare professional?

Preserving human dignity through narrative care

In this chapter, I have argued for an understanding of storytelling practice in palliative care as a possible way of upholding or preserving the dignity of identity. As Nordenfelt

(2004) stresses, the dignity of identity is vulnerable and can be under particular threat, or can even be lost due to the threat of serious illness. One of the crucial aspects of dignity of identity is that it relates to us as 'persons with a history and persons with a future with all our relationships to other human beings' (Nordenfelt 2004, p. 75). As I have shown in the stories of illness, a narrative understanding can offer an interpretation that can bring a sense of continuity to the breakdown that the illness represents – continuity of the past and the present, as well as of the present and the future.

At the same time, I have argued that stories where illness is absent (such as stories of everyday life and the past) can also bring a sense of continuity, contributing to dignity of identity by providing versions of a still-functioning everyday life, as well as a presentation and confirmation of one's past life, supporting who one was and still is. But this chapter has also shown that a narrative interpretation or narrative identity is as vulnerable as a person's dignity of identity. Stories of illness can break down and, as we have seen, some of the narrators chose not to talk about their illness at all.

Storytelling always involves presenting one version among many. As Donald Spence (1982) argues, there is a difference between 'historical truth' and 'narrative truth'. Narrative is related to meaning-making through a reconstruction of reality, where the aim is 'to turn the patient's life into a meaningful story' (Spence 1982, p. 158). The different stories show how one can sustain a version of a dignity of identity through the act of storytelling. The stories that I have gathered in my work with palliative care patients have shown great variety in what the patients wanted to discuss. By giving them an opportunity to share what was important to them, the various stories show how different narrative truths can be important ways of establishing continuity in difficult life situations.

This way of looking at the stories implies an understanding of care as *narrative care* (Kenyon, Bohlmeijer & Randall 2010). Stories constitute narrative care because the self is formed through the act of storytelling. Furthermore, storytelling implies a double affirmation. The first affirmation is the relationship between the narrator and the listener that stories require, which gives the narrator an audience for their story. The second affirmation is the narrator's confirmation of themselves: I am still here with my illness, but also with my stories, my memories, my relationships – and with a voice.

The act of storytelling should not be seen as a 'quick fix' or a naïve solution to the fragility and vulnerability of terminally ill patients. As I have experienced in my narrative practice with palliative care patients, storytelling is a fragile enterprise. But, at the same time, storytelling is a meaning-making process that can remain vital until the end of life. According to Frank (1995), one of the goals of narrative ethics is restoring a sense of agency to ill people. Attending to the stories of patients equips them with resources that can, at least to some degree, preserve important aspects of their dignity and identity, both by giving them an opportunity to experience their situation in various ways and by giving them an audience that will affirm their experiences, worries, dreams and thoughts.

Chapter summary

- Patients' narratives are related to both identity and dignity.
- Narrative care acknowledges the need to listen and honour the meaning that ill people are trying to construct through storytelling.
- The act of storytelling implies a double affirmation: on the one hand, storytelling involves a listener who acknowledges the story and the teller; on the other hand, the telling gives the storyteller confirmation of themselves.

Suggested reading

For more in-depth understanding, you are encouraged to read:

Frank, A.W. (1995). *The wounded storyteller: body, illness, and ethics*. Chicago: University of Chicago Press.

Nordenfelt, L. & Edgar, A. (2005). The four notions of dignity. *Quality in Ageing*. **6**(1), 17–21.

Synnes, O. (2015). Narratives of nostalgia in the face of death: the importance of lighter stories of the past in palliative care. *Journal of Aging Studies*. **34**, 169–76.

References

Broyard, A. (1992). *Intoxicated by my illness: and other writings on life and death*. New York: Ballantine Books.

Bury, M. (1982). Chronic illness as biographical disruption. *Sociology of Health & Illness*. **4**, 167–82.

Charmaz, K. (1983). Loss of self: a fundamental form of suffering in the chronically ill. *Sociology of Health & Illness*. **5**: 168–95.

Charon, R. (2006). *Narrative medicine: honoring the stories of illness*. Oxford: Oxford University Press.

Davis, F. (1979). *Yearning for yesterday: a sociology of nostalgia*. New York: The Free Press.

Deciu Ritivoi, A. (2002). *Yesterday's self: nostalgia and the immigrant identity*. Oxford: Rowman & Littlefield.

Deciu Ritivoi, A. (2008). 'Identity and narrative' in D. Herman, M. Jahn & M.-L. Ryan (eds) *Routledge encyclopedia of narrative theory*. London: Routledge, 231–35.

Edwards, P. (2005). An overview of the end-of-life discussion. *International Journal of Palliative Nursing*. **11**, 21–27.

Frank, A.W. (1995). *The wounded storyteller: body, illness, and ethics*. Chicago: University of Chicago Press.

Frank, A.W. (1998). Just listening: narrative and deep illness. *Families, Systems, & Health*. **16**, 197–212.

Frank, A.W. (2010). *Letting stories breathe: a socio-narratology*. Chicago: University of Chicago Press.

Giddens, A. (1991). *Modernity and self-identity: self and society in the late modern age*. Cambridge: Polity Press.

Gunaratnam, Y. & Oliviere, D. (2009). *Narrative and stories in health care: illness, dying, and bereavement*. New York: Oxford University Press.

Kenyon, G., Bohlmeijer, E. & Randall, W. (eds) (2011). *Storying later life: issues, investigations, and interventions in narrative care*. New York: Oxford University Press.

Kvåle, K. (2007). Do cancer patients always want to talk about difficult emotions? A qualitative study of cancer inpatients' communication needs. *European Journal of Oncology Nursing*. **11**, 320–27.

MacIntyre, A. (2007). *After virtue: a study in moral theory*. London: Duckworth.

Mattingly, C. (1998). *Healing dramas and clinical plots: the narrative structure of experience*. Cambridge: Cambridge University Press.

Murray, D. (2002). *Faith in hospices: spiritual care and the end of life*. London: SPCK Publishing.

Nolan, S. (2011). *Spiritual care at the end of life: the chaplain as a 'hopeful presence'*. London: Jessica Kingsley Publishers.

Nordenfelt, L. (2004). The varieties of dignity. *Health Care Analysis*. **12**(2), 69–81.

Nordenfelt, L. & Edgar, A. (2005). The four notions of dignity. *Quality in Ageing*. **6**(1), 17–21.

Ragan, S.L., Wittenberg, E. & Hall, H.T. (2003). The communication of palliative care for the elderly cancer patient. *Health Commun. 15*, 219–26.

Ricoeur, P. (1976). *Interpretation theory: discourse and the surplus of meaning*. Fort Worth, Texas: Texas Christian University Press.

Ricoeur, P. (1988). *Time and narrative,* Volume 3. Chicago: University of Chicago Press.

Ricoeur, P. (1992). *Oneself as another*. Chicago: University of Chicago Press.

Routledge, C., Arndt, J., Wildschut, T., Sedikides, C., & Hart, C.M. (2011). The past makes the present meaningful: nostalgia as an existential resource. *Journal of Personality and Social Psychology*. **101**(3), 638–52.

Rybarczyk, B. & Bellg, A. (1997). *Listening to life stories: a new approach to stress intervention in health care.* New York: Springer.

Saunders, C. (1996). A personal therapeutic journey. *British Medical Journal.* **313**, 1599–1601.

Saunders, C. (2001). The evolution of palliative care. *Journal of the Royal Society of Medicine.* **94**, 430–32.

Saunders, C. (2003). *Watch with me: inspiration for a life in hospice care.* Sheffield: Mortal Press.

Spence, D. (1982). *Narrative truth and historical truth: meaning and interpretation in psychoanalysis.* New York: W.W. Norton.

Synnes, O. (2012). *Forteljing som identitetskonstruksjon ved alvorleg sjukdom: ein hermeneutisk analyse av alvorleg sjuke og døyande sine forteljingar [Narrative as identity construction in serious illness: a hermeneutic analysis of stories of terminally ill patients].* PhD thesis. Oslo: Norwegian School of Theology.

Synnes, O. (2015). Narratives of nostalgia in the face of death: the importance of lighter stories of the past in palliative care. *Journal of Aging Studies.* **34**, 169–76.

Taylor C. (1989). *Sources of the self: the making of the modern identity.* Cambridge: Cambridge University Press.

Thomas, C., Reeve, J., Bingley, A., Brown, J., Payne, S., & Lynch, T. (2009). Narrative research methods in palliative care contexts: two case studies. *Journal of Pain Symptom Management.* **37**, 788–96.

Thulesius, H., Hakansson, A., & Petersson, K. (2003). Balancing: a basic process in end-of-life cancer care. *Qualitative Health Research.* **13**, 1353–77.

Wikan, U. (2000). 'With life in one's lap: the story of an eye/I (or two)' in C. Mattingly & L.C. Garro (eds) *Narrative and the cultural construction of illness and healing.* Berkeley: University of California Press. pp. 212–36.

Williams, G. (1984). The genesis of chronic illness: narrative re-construction. *Sociology of Health & Illness.* **6**, 175–200.

Chapter 6

Reintegrating spirituality and dignity in nursing and healthcare: a relational model of practice

Wilfred McSherry

Introduction

The last few decades have witnessed the introduction of many slogans or phrases describing the goal of nursing or healthcare. These have included, for instance, 'holistic care', 'individualised care', 'spiritual care', 'dignity in care', 'person-centred care' and, more recently, 'compassionate care'. The common denominator in all these terms is that they seek to combat the prevailing medical/scientific model which has infiltrated and fragmented the delivery of care. More recently, these slogans seem to have been increasingly used in response to media reports claiming (especially in the UK) that nurses lack compassion and care. These phrases appear to offer an altruistic, humanistic view of individuals, highlighting the more subjective, sensitive and arguably contentious elements of nursing such as spirituality and dignity.

This chapter therefore explores the relationship between spirituality and dignity, demonstrating how the symbiotic nature of these concepts is fundamental and central in the provision of person-centred care and ultimately in delivering high-quality compassionate nursing and healthcare.

To illustrate the importance of these concepts, I draw upon a professional narrative (which could be termed 'a critical incident') that ignited my interest in spirituality and, more recently, dignity in care. This professional narrative shows how these two interrelated and interdependent concepts are central to the delivery of nursing and healthcare and, fundamentally, to preserving the dignity of the individual. The works of several authors in the fields of spirituality (Howden 1992, Reed 1992, Clarke 2013) and dignity (Fenton & Mitchell 2002, Nordenfelt & Edgar 2005, Jacobson 2009) are utilised to illuminate the importance of these concepts for nursing and healthcare practice.

Finally, a relational model of nursing is presented, demonstrating the central significance of dignity and spirituality in the delivery of nursing care and how these concepts influence individual and organisational values and cultures and, ultimately, the quality of care provided.

Learning objectives

This chapter will enable you to:

- Demonstrate how altruistic and humanistic aspects of the person, such as spirituality and dignity, are central to nursing and healthcare.
- Highlight the fact that dignity and spirituality are central to the identity of the person, thereby influencing the values, attitudes, behaviour and practice of healthcare professionals.
- Reinforce these concepts as fundamental aspects of caring and compassionate care, which are integral to the concept of holistic practice.
- Provide a relational model of spirituality and dignity to guide and inform nursing and healthcare practice.

Background: the evolution of nursing

Nursing is a relatively new profession (in comparison to – say – medicine) and it continues to evolve, develop, respond and *adapt* to meet the holistic and person-centred needs of people across the world, meaning that nursing is a universal activity. 'Adapt' is printed in italics here because it is an important word, since present-day nursing clearly relies more upon scientific, digital and social technologies than nursing did in the past. This development reinforces the evolutionary nature of nursing and the need for the profession to be responsive to the changing needs of society, adopting and utilising new knowledge, skills, technologies and practices as they emerge.

Yet, despite its transient nature and the need for nurses to adapt, it can be argued that the precise nature of nursing stays unchanged, in that it transcends time and remains a constant in the 'milieu of change'. In order to understand this, we need to explore what we mean by nursing. The most seminal definition is the one provided by Virginia Henderson (1964, p. 63), which reads:

> The unique function of the nurse is to assist the individual, sick or well, in the performance of those activities contributing to health or its recovery (or to a peaceful death) that he would perform unaided if he had the necessary strength, will or knowledge; and to do this in such a way as to help him gain independence as rapidly as possible.

This definition articulates quite clearly that 'the individual' with all their diverse and 'holistic' needs (the recipient of nursing) is the central focus of all nursing care and activity. Therefore, it could be argued that, despite all the advances in the art and science of nursing, the essence of nursing remains unchanged. Henderson's (1964) definition of nursing is as relevant today as when it was first published five decades ago. Furthermore, a more contemporary definition of nursing, produced by the Royal College of Nursing (RCN 2014, p. 3), affirms that certain characteristics of nursing practice transcend time and remain constant:

> The use of clinical judgement in the provision of care to enable people to improve, maintain, or recover health, to cope with health problems, and to achieve the best possible quality of life, whatever their disease or disability, until death.

A common theme in both definitions is the individual: the person at the centre of all nursing practice, intervention and activity. Furthermore, the use of the word 'clinical' in the RCN definition suggests infiltration from the medical model of care. Although not explicit in either definition, nursing activity should always preserve the dignity of each person. Again, the way to achieve this is through a holistic, person-centred approach.

Interestingly, the definition offered by the International Council of Nurses (ICN 2014) broadens the scope and practice of nursing by embracing other important roles, such as health promotion and prevention, research and management. Yet the individual, irrespective of their position on the lifespan trajectory, remains at the centre of all nursing activity:

> Nursing encompasses autonomous and collaborative care of individuals of all ages, families, groups and communities, sick or well and in all settings. Nursing includes the promotion of health, prevention of illness, and the care of ill, disabled and dying people. Advocacy, promotion of a safe environment, research, participation in shaping health policy and in patient and health systems management, and education are also key nursing roles.

An analysis of the ICN Code of Ethics (2012, p. 1) offers further description of nursing, stressing the importance of some key dimensions:

> Nurses have four fundamental responsibilities: to promote health, to prevent illness, to restore health and to alleviate suffering. The need for nursing is universal.
>
> Inherent in nursing is a respect for human rights, including cultural rights, the right to life and choice, to dignity and to be treated with respect. Nursing care is respectful of and unrestricted by considerations of age, colour, creed, culture, disability or illness, gender, sexual orientation, nationality, politics, race or social status.

Notably, the words 'spiritual' and 'dignity' are each used twice in the entire document, thus affirming that that they *do* have a place in nursing care.

The spiritual aspects of nursing

Bradshaw (1994, p. 169) writes: 'The spiritual dimension in nursing's tradition cannot be separated from the history of nursing itself.' This quotation emphasises the importance of nursing history and heritage, indicating that these are important considerations for the ongoing development of the profession. Bradshaw (1994) thus reinforces the centrality of the spiritual dimension as a founding principle and value on which the whole nursing profession is based. This raises a crucial question: what happens when healthcare generally and nursing in particular remove the spiritual dimension from practice? In reality, this question implies that nursing can reject and ignore the spiritual legacy from which it emerged. Before we can answer it, there is a need to say something very briefly about the spiritual and historical evolution of nursing and the philosophies and ideologies that have shaped, and continue to shape, nursing practice.

Until the formal regulation of the nursing profession, much of what we call 'nursing' was carried out by religious organisations and institutions (Narayanasamy 2001) and, indeed, ordinary women in the course of their everyday obligations. The preface of Florence Nightingale's (1969, p. 3) *Notes on Nursing* reinforces this point: 'They [*Notes on Nursing*] are meant simply to give hints for thought to women who have personal charge of the health of others. … every woman is a nurse.' Hence nursing and caring were not the preserve of a social elite. Instead, these skills were practised by women of every race, creed, colour and class, both secular and religious, throughout society.

Furthermore, nursing and caring was not just concerned with alleviating human suffering but with the general health and wellbeing of all people – especially those [women] with personal charge of others. This implies that nursing and caring were about supporting the individual not just physically but socially, psychologically and spiritually. Although words such as 'dignity' and 'spirituality' are not used, there is a realisation by Nightingale (1969) that caring is about being responsive to the 'holistic' needs of those in your charge.

Dignity in care

Whitehead and Wheeler (2008a, 2008b) provide a useful review of the concepts of privacy and dignity. They affirm that interest in these concepts in the UK started in the 1960s in the field of psychiatry, and then extended into hospitals and other areas during the 1990s. Therefore, 'dignity in care' is not necessarily a new concept. Furthermore, the study undertaken by Whitehead and Wheeler in 2008 indicates that there is global interest in the idea of 'dignity in care', perhaps partly due to a realisation that dignity is a universal and fundamental human need. But if the importance of dignity in care is globally recognised, why is there a growing movement campaigning for dignity in nursing and healthcare? As indicated earlier, one of the drivers for this movement is the increasing influence of medical and biological model of care and other prevailing values, ideologies and economic, financial and bureaucratic models, which detract from the caring environment and impede the preservation of human dignity.

The medical model of care

Discussing the medical model of care, Pearson, Vaughan and Fitzgerald (2005, p. 44) state:

> In this model people are seen as biological beings, made up of cells, which then make tissues, which then make organs, which then make systems. All of these interact and communicate with each other to achieve harmony or balance, a state called homeostasis.

Not everything about the medical model is negative or bad. On the contrary, many diseases have been eradicated from the world by utilising the medical model, which has offered pioneering treatments and alleviated immense suffering. However, interestingly, an old *Churchill Livingstone's Dictionary of Nursing* (1996, p. 228) comments that the use of the term 'the medical model' in a nursing context 'signifies that the focus of nursing is the medical diagnosis allocated by the doctor'.

My concern about adopting a purely medical and reductionist model of care in nursing is that this approach can render the individual person invisible. It could be argued that nursing has become more medically focused over the past 20 years; and we have consequently lost sight of our unique selling point – what we, as nurses, bring to healthcare in terms of care and caring. This reductionist approach has left a gap at the heart of nursing – and perhaps helps to explain the growing interest in the areas of spirituality and dignity, in order to preserve a more person-centred approach to care.

Theories of spirituality and dignity

This section explores some of the theoretical attributes associated with the concepts of spirituality and dignity. As outlined earlier, during the past two decades there has been a growing awareness of the importance of these ideas in the provision of nursing and healthcare. However, it is all too easy to assume that spirituality and dignity are unrelated, independent concepts, when – in reality – they are deeply interrelated and interdependent. We cannot conserve any person's dignity if we fail to acknowledge and support their spiritual aspects. Therefore, it is a grave misconception to separate spirituality and dignity from one another.

The way we assess, plan, implement and evaluate aspects of spiritual care depends upon how we define an individual – and the role that spirituality plays in their life and how this contributes to their individual identity and sense of health and wellbeing. To preserve someone's dignity is to validate them as an individual, appreciating their uniqueness. It also means understanding that we confer, maintain and affirm the person's dignity through communication. To achieve this in everyday practice, we must accept that the spiritual aspects of care are often inseparable from good fundamental nursing and healthcare practice (Clarke 2013).

Yet, in order to identify the spiritual within the greater 'whole' of nursing and healthcare practice, we also need to explore its constituent parts and attributes. There are numerous definitions of spirituality within the nursing and healthcare literature (see Table 6.1).

Table 6.1
Definitions of spirituality in healthcare spanning the last two decades

Author(s)	Definition
Stoll (1989, p. 6)	'Spirituality is my being; my inner person. It is who I am – unique and alive. It is me expressed through my body, my thinking, my feelings, my judgments, and my creativity. My spirituality motivates me to choose meaningful relationships and pursuits. Through my spirituality I give and receive love; I respond to and appreciate God, other people, a sunset, a symphony, and spring. I am driven forward, sometimes because of pain, sometimes in spite of pain. Spirituality allows me to reflect on myself. I am a person because of my spirituality – motivated and enabled to value, to worship, and to communicate with the holy, the transcendent.'
Murray & Zentner (1989, p. 259)	'A quality that goes beyond religious affiliation that strives for inspirations, reverence, awe, meaning and purpose, even in those who do not believe in any good. The spiritual dimension tries to be in harmony with the universe, and strives for answers about the infinite, and comes into focus when the person faces emotional stress, physical illness or death.'
Males & Boswell (1990, p. 35)	'It is not easy to define spirituality since it concerns the way in which men and women may understand their existence and the action which comes from an understanding; the knowledge of things both within an individual and of the existence and importance of things beyond him or her. It is important to point out this knowledge is not the grasp of intellectual facts but rather a reverence for mysteries of life which no-one can fully understand. It is not, therefore, something which can be regarded as being unattainable for people with learning difficulties.'

Reed (1992, p. 350)	'Specifically spirituality refers to the propensity to make meaning through a sense of relatedness to dimensions that transcend the self in such a way that empowers and does not devalue the individual. This relatedness may be experienced intrapersonally (as a connectedness within oneself), interpersonally (in the context of others and the natural environment) and transpersonally (referring to a sense of relatedness to the unseen, God, or power greater than the self and ordinary source).'
Tanyi (2002, p. 506)	'Spirituality is a personal search for meaning and purpose in life, which may or may not be related to religion. It entails connection to self-chosen and/or religious beliefs, values and practices that give meaning to life, thereby inspiring and motivating individuals to achieve their optimal being. This connection brings faith, hope, peace, and empowerment. The results are joy, forgiveness of oneself and others, awareness and acceptance of hardship and mortality, a heightened sense of physical and emotional well-being, and the ability to transcend beyond the infirmities of existence.'

Inherent in all the definitions in Table 6.1 is the relationship between dignity and spirituality. The definitions reveal that the concept of spirituality is intimately bound up with dignity and an individual's sense of identity: how they see and feel about themselves and their place in the world.

Analysis of these definitions reveals that spirituality is often predicated on the following essential attributes:

- Existentialism: the way individuals derive and find meaning, purpose and fulfilment in life.
- Relationship: the relationships that are significant to an individual's sense of identity, health and wellbeing – these could be relationships with family, friends, the environment, community and/or creatures.
- Transcendence: a sense of something greater and beyond the self – this could be God, a deity, supreme being or Higher Power. It could also be aspects of life that enable the individual to transcend themselves or particular situations.
- Connection: the sense of connection that individuals have with others, with the environment and with God or some Higher Power.
- Religiosity: for some people their spirituality and worldview are based upon adherence to a specific religious teaching, doctrine or practice. This adherence informs and influences their beliefs, attitudes, values and behaviour.

This list of essential attributes of spirituality demonstrates that spirituality may be very individually focused for some people, while for others it is expressed through a sense of community. This list also shows that spirituality is broad, complex and deeply subjective, which may help to explain why so many different models and theories addressing this concept are emerging within nursing and healthcare. According to Reed (1992, see Table 6.1), spirituality is concerned with the issue of transcendence. This suggests that spirituality is concerned with the individual and their relationship with others and the environment. This author also reaffirms the notion that spirituality involves awareness of something greater or beyond oneself (the mystical nature inherent in every individual). Meanwhile Howden (1992), through the development of the Spiritual Assessment Scale, validates the notion that spirituality is a multifaceted dimension embracing Purpose or Meaning, Innerness, Interconnectedness and Transcendence. Again, the interconnectedness and interdependence between all these attributes suggests they have a close connection to aspects of human dignity. In other words, for nurses or healthcare professionals to deny the existence of such aspects of the person may lead to a violation of their dignity.

The aforementioned theories imply that spirituality and spiritual care can be intimately intertwined with the everyday practice of nursing and healthcare. This may make it hard to pinpoint exactly what is spiritual care (as opposed to good fundamental care) that is truly holistic and person-centred. Interestingly, Clarke (2009, 2013) offers a more practical and applied approach by suggesting that spiritual care is integral to nursing practice. In her view, spiritual care is not something additional but something that is experienced and manifested in the delivery of everyday nursing care. Clarke (2013, p. 193) illustrates this wonderfully in the following:

> Hopefully my inadequate voice will inspire others to take this vision and to develop ever more creative ways to explore the true relationship between spirituality and nursing – not only to develop spiritual care, because that would be a very limited goal, but rather to use the concept of making all care spiritual to develop and improve everything that nurses do.

As one of the proponents of spirituality in healthcare (McSherry 2006, 2007), I have been criticised by colleagues for not providing a clear conceptual or operational definition of the concept. These criticisms are unpublished voices but their responses do still highlight a significant omission. However, this omission has been deliberate on my part, as I don't think this concept can be adequately defined in words. Nor do I think that the spiritual aspects of life can be contained or captured in a box.

Similarly, Narayanasamy (2001) says that there is no such thing as an authoritative definition of spirituality and this is reinforced by Swinton and Pattison (2010, p. 236), who write: 'As a matter of fact, it is probably important that spirituality remains a contested and functional concept rather than becoming consolidated ...' This implies that there is room to explore and develop the concept. We need to ensure that it is not constrained by definitions and boundaries or, indeed, arguments about relevance and suitability. It is clear that spirituality as a concept, and perhaps as a field of scientific study, is still very much in its infancy. Therefore, there is a need for ongoing exploration and development. The fact that the concept is still being 'contested' and debated will allow a rich dialogue to continue, enabling understanding to evolve. This will ensure that the concept's functional elements are fully explored, and it is not constructed and consolidated prematurely.

With regard to definition and understanding, I developed a definition of spirituality for use in my inaugural professorial lecture in April 2009, which was cited in McSherry and Smith (2012, p. 118). This definition is not superior in any way to those already referred to in this chapter; on the contrary. However, I have sought to highlight the relationship between spirituality and dignity:

> Spirituality is universal, deeply personal and individual; it goes beyond formal notions of ritual or religious practice to encompass the unique capacity of each individual. It is at the core and essence of who we are, that spark which permeates the entire fabric of the person and demands that we are all worthy of dignity and respect. It transcends intellectual capability, elevating the status of all of humanity to that of the sacred.

This definition was based upon and derived from personal experience, reflection and analysis of the empirical work I had undertaken over almost two decades. It also reflected some of the themes emerging in the existing literature. It provides a description of those attributes that are fundamental to spirituality. For me, spirituality is not an intellectual activity; it is central to identity and dignity and therefore relevant to all people. Crucially, dignity and spirituality are interdependent, since nurses and healthcare professionals cannot preserve a person's dignity if they do not address their religious, spiritual and personal belief. To ignore or neglect these aspects of the person, for whatever reason, is to fail to see them holistically and comprehensively. Furthermore, such omissions may lead to a violation of that person's dignity.

The importance of dignity

Dignity – just like spirituality – is a subjective concept, and the way it is perceived and received in practice is individually determined and experienced. Therefore, an action that may preserve one person's dignity may lead to a violation of another's.

For the purposes of this chapter, the work of the following are used to highlight the importance of dignity in a therapeutic and caring environment. The four-notion model of dignity constructed by Nordenfelt and Edgar (2005) and the pioneering taxonomy of Nora Jacobson (2009) are utilised to illustrate key points in the professional narrative presented below. In addition, the Attitudes (A), Behaviour (B), Compassionate (C), and Dialogue (D) of dignity conserving care model created by Harvey Max Chochinov (2007) have informed thinking about and the development of the relational model.

After undertaking a concept analysis of dignity in the context of caring for older people, Fenton and Mitchell (2002, p. 21) constructed the following definition:

> Dignity is a state of physical, emotional and spiritual comfort, with each individual valued for his or her uniqueness and his or her individuality celebrated. Dignity is promoted when individuals are enabled to do the best within their capabilities, exercise control, make choices and feel involved in the decision-making that underpins their care.

This definition demonstrates the symbiotic and integral relationship that dignity and spirituality share and the importance of these concepts in the provision of individualised, person-centred and holistic healthcare. The definition affirms that dignity is about preserving an individual's sense of autonomy and independence by enabling them to exercise choice and control. The definition also implies that if those working in healthcare do not preserve the uniqueness of each person and enable people to fulfil their potential, this could lead to a violation of dignity. In other words, certain attitudes, behaviours and practices can either preserve or violate dignity.

The four notions of dignity

As part of a wider European project, Nordenfelt and Edgar (2005) developed a useful model of dignity, involving four notions: 'absolute dignity' (*Menschenwürde*), 'dignity as merit', 'dignity of moral stature' and 'dignity of personal identity' (see p. 7).

Analysis of Nordenfelt's and Edgar's (2005) model indicates that we understand dignity on different levels. On one level, dignity is 'absolute' – something 'sacred' and 'infinite' that cannot be stolen or removed from a person through violation or degradation. The second level of dignity may be called 'social dignity' or 'relative dignity', since it is influenced by external factors that affect the person both extrinsically and intrinsically, such as attitudes, language, behaviour, cultures and environments. However, it must be stressed that, while these factors may violate the person's social dignity, they can never remove the absolute dignity that comes from their humanity. This is not to say that individuals will not feel wounded, hurt and offended by such violations, which are often painful, damaging and have a detrimental impact on the individual's sense of self and identity. They can also powerfully affect the way a specific individual, team or organisation is viewed by the recipient of such violation(s).

The notions of dignity preservation and violation are certainly fundamental to the work of Jacobson (2009). From her qualitative research with marginal and vulnerable groups, she developed her dignity taxonomy. This taxonomy offers valuable insights into the attitudes, behaviours and actions that can preserve a person's dignity such as acceptance, creativity, empowerment and courtesy; and, conversely, those that can violate dignity such as rudeness, objectification, intrusion and bullying.

Frequently used terms in nursing

As stated earlier, nursing and healthcare have witnessed the introduction of a number of catchphrases or slogans over the last few decades. These have included:

- Individualised care
- Holistic care
- Spiritual care
- Dignity in care
- Person-centred care
- Integrated care
- Evidence-based care
- Compassionate care
- Integrated care.

As stated earlier, the common denominator in all these terms is that they seek to combat the prevailing medical and scientific model that has infiltrated and fragmented nursing care. These phrases seem to offer a more altruistic and humanistic view of individuals, highlighting the more subjective, sensitive and (arguably) contentious elements of nursing such as spirituality. Perhaps the primary reason why we constantly create these slogans is to ensure that the main focus stays upon the individual who is receiving care. Deviating from this primary purpose and pursuing other goals (including political and bureaucratic agendas) can have catastrophic consequences for the public and, indeed, for those providing care.

What happens when we lose sight of the person?

As outlined in Chapter 1, a number of damning reports have been published in the UK (The Patients Association, 2009, 2010, 2011, the Parliamentary and Health Service Ombudsman (2011, 2015), criticising nurses and healthcare professionals for a lack of compassion and care. These accusations reached a deafening crescendo in *The Report of the Mid Staffordshire NHS Foundation Trust Public Inquiry* (2013), which highlighted significant failings and neglect in care that allegedly led to the death of over 400 patients. Collectively, these reports reveal the factors that can cause organisations to lose sight of the importance of the person (be this the patient, public or staff) – for example, poor organisational cultures, attitudes, values and systems that dehumanise and violate human dignity. All these reports show that organisations providing care should regularly evaluate and review the values that inform, influence and shape their culture.

My professional narrative on spirituality and dignity in care

I am constantly asked what originally ignited my interest in the areas of spirituality and dignity. The following is a personal and professional narrative about what led me to explore, develop and 'champion' the more humanistic values of nursing and healthcare revealed in all the aforementioned reports. This narrative demonstrates the importance of reflection, supervision and, above all, action that leads to change.

The following narrative (taken from McSherry 2006) describes an incident that has had a huge influence on me as a person and as a nurse. This 'critical incident' had such a profound impact upon me all those years ago that it remains the driving force behind everything I have tried to achieve in the development of nursing and healthcare practice and education. This narrative reinforces the point that spirituality and (by default) dignity are not separate isolated concepts but are interrelated and interdependent, meaning we cannot have one without the other.

Let me start by setting the scene: I was a newly qualified staff nurse working on a busy medical ward. I had been qualified for about eight weeks. Having had some days off, I arrived for the late shift and the following occurred:

> Peter, 72 years old, was known by his family and friends to like a drink or two. He was admitted to hospital with an acute episode of chest pain. A diagnosis of angina was made, since ECGs showed no evidence of recent infarct.
>
> It came to light later that Peter was a practising Roman Catholic who found meaning and purpose in his beliefs. Peter had only been in hospital overnight and he had not seen his wife because she had taken herself off to their daughters 'down south' after an argument. Nevertheless, she was informed by Peter of his admission into hospital and she was intending to visit as soon as possible. In the afternoon on the following day Peter was due to be discharged when he developed sudden severe central chest pain, collapsing with a cardiac arrest – resuscitation was initiated. During the resuscitation Peter's wife arrived on the ward. Unfortunately, she did not see Peter before he died. After Peter's death his wife asked if the Catholic priest had been. Inspection of the nursing notes showed that nothing in relation to religion had been entered.
>
> Let me elaborate a little further...
>
> As indicated, I was newly qualified and was working on a busy medical ward: the old Nightingale style of ward. I had been on my days off and came onto a late shift and was in handover. The nurse in charge allocated me my patients and after report I went out to introduce myself to all the patients on the ward as was my approach. I came to Peter, he asked me to put his outdoor clothes on the bed and to draw the curtains around his bed. I left him to see the other patients.

Something drew me back to the curtain. I found Peter collapsed across his bed. I felt for a pulse. It was very slow – something like 15 beats per minute. I pulled the emergency button and a 'Crash call' was put out. The team arrived on the ward.

My role, being a newly qualified nurse, was to bring equipment and drugs for the team. I was asked to bring a particular drug from the cupboard when a lady approached me and said she had come to collect Peter. I informed the lady (who I learned was Peter's wife) that the doctors were with her husband. I showed her to the dayroom and indicated that I would come back as soon as I had some information. As I left she said quite insistently, 'I need to see my husband!' I went back to the registrar leading the resuscitation and asked if Peter's wife could come and see her husband, as I was aware that he was still fluctuating in and out of consciousness. I was met with a firm 'No' and another couple of expletives.

As I was walking towards the dayroom I thought to myself 'Four years at university doesn't prepare you for this.' I went back into the dayroom and I forget what I said. But again, as I left, I was met with the same request but this time more firmly. Just as I was about to ask again whether Peter's wife could see him, she lunged forward and said, 'Who the bloody hell are you to tell me I can't see my husband?'. Her protests were quickly ushered away by the charge nurse and senior nursing staff.

Peter went on to have a full cardiac arrest and unfortunately died. The registrar said, 'Wilf, you can come with me when I break the bad news!' It was like walking into a war zone – the hostility, anger, anxiety and the sadness felt were overwhelming. Peter's wife was distraught and very frustrated by her exclusion, however well this had been intended. During the conversation, Peter's wife asked, 'Where is the priest?' I thought 'priest?' – no patients had ever asked for a priest during my four years of nurse training. So as not to compound the situation, I sneaked out while the registrar was still talking to look at the nursing notes. Nothing had been written or documented indicating what religion Peter was. I therefore had to go back and ask what type of priest (Roman Catholic, Anglican, etc), adding to the frustration and distress.

The situation was made worse when the switchboard informed me that the Roman Catholic chaplain was away at a Conference. The ecumenical chaplain came to offer support and I spent almost 50 minutes locating a local priest to come to the ward.

I first met Peter at around 13.30 pm and his wife left the ward at around 19.00 pm. Over six hours were spent offering support and care. Even now, as I recall this event, I can see Peter's wife walking away from the ward, and her sadness and grief are still all too evident. There was a catalogue of issues around lack of assessment and poor documentation – what we now consider to be important elements of care.

What did I learn?

I learned many lessons from this incident. It taught me to be reflective and to challenge – not in a dogmatic or aggressive manner but as a critical friend asking questions. This is a practice I still believe in today because change and innovation never occur without question and challenge. This event also indicated to me that nurses and healthcare professionals must remember that individuals are not just a conglomeration of physical systems and parts; we are all living beings with a whole range of personal beliefs, values and emotional and psychological needs that shape our dignity and identity and uniqueness. This incident highlighted the importance of paying equal attention to other often-neglected dimensions of each person, such as their religious, personal or spiritual beliefs.

In healthcare we seem to have adopted an increasingly scientific/medical approach. The team were technically competent and their practice and intervention could not be challenged, as they did everything possible to preserve Peter's life. Yet the danger of adopting a solely scientific approach is that we fail to look at the other practical or humanistic dimensions, such as the effect a person's personal, religious and spiritual beliefs have upon their human dignity and sense of identity, as outlined in the model developed by Nordenfelt and Edgar (2005).

Therefore, while the team did well in the scientific aspects of care, we didn't do so well in others. We did not address and support Peter's religious beliefs and spiritual practices, and we did not listen to his needs or those of his wife. These professional attitudes and behaviours, however well intended, led to a violation of dignity. In hindsight, it is easy to reflect upon this situation in the light of Jacobson's (2009) dignity taxonomy and identify those attitudes, behaviours and practices that contributed to the violation. However, it is often harder for individuals, teams and organisations to reflect constructively on such incidents, identifying what could have been done differently to preserve the dignity of all involved.

It is my belief that we cannot provide dignified care unless the spiritual dimension is included and addressed. This position is echoed in the definition provided by Fenton and Mitchell (2002). Unless nurses and healthcare professionals address the spiritual dimension, we fail to recognise and support the uniqueness of each individual and the preservation of their dignity.

> **Critical thinking activities**
> 1 How would you have responded if you had found yourself in the situation outlined in the narrative?
> 2 What was the most important lesson for you, having read the narrative?
> 3 Which caring or nursing theory would you choose to help you interpret or better understand the narrative?

Relational model of spirituality and dignity in nursing and healthcare practice

In this section I offer a relational model for nursing and healthcare practice that demonstrates the importance of re-integrating spirituality and dignity. Recent reports outlined earlier, and published in the UK, have emphasised the need for nursing and healthcare to look again at the types of values they adopt when delivering patient care. The implications of these reports extend globally, since they suggest that some nurses and healthcare organisations are failing to recognise the uniqueness of the individual. This may be partly due to systemic failure, the reasons for which are numerous and complex. However, the net result is that the general public feel that these failings have had a significant and detrimental impact on the ability of these organisations to provide safe, good-quality care.

I use the word 're-integrating' because it is my opinion that spirituality and dignity are still present in nursing and healthcare but the importance of their contribution has, to some degree, been devalued and lost. The concepts still exist but they have somehow been misplaced (eroded, neglected and forgotten) and this means that nurses and healthcare professionals must find ways of re-integrating and re-engaging with them so that they become more visible and prominent in care delivery. In this way, their unique contribution to the quality of care can be identified and, importantly, celebrated.

Spirituality and dignity are not competing forces, since both shape the identity of the individual, influencing attitudes, beliefs and ultimately our actions and approach to nursing care. This is shown in Figure 6.1 (below), which illustrates a relational model of nursing and healthcare.

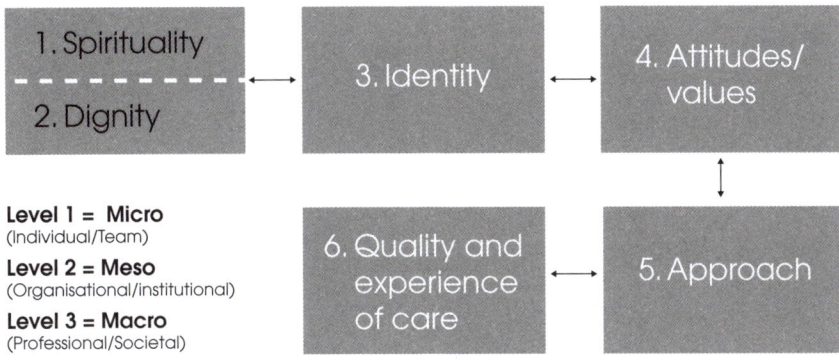

Figure 6.1 Relational model of nursing and healthcare

As demonstrated earlier, nursing has a clear foundation, history and evolution and these determine the knowledge and skills nurses require in order to provide safe, high-quality care. It could be argued that what constitutes safe and high-quality care keeps changing, since the art and science of nursing are continually progressing and evolving. This is important because it is all too easy to look back at nursing and healthcare practice with a sense of nostalgia and assume that everything was good or, conversely, bad. For example, if we look at the way many older people living with dementia were cared for in institutions in the late 1970s and early 1980s, there was an overuse of physical restraints, tranquillisers and sedatives to control challenging behaviour. These are now considered bad practice or, in some cases, outlawed because they are seen as depriving the person of their liberty. In this sense, the way we care for people living with dementia has changed beyond recognition and this has been achieved through greater understanding, research and education.

The definitions of nursing presented earlier affirm that nursing is a dynamic profession that responds to the changing needs of people and society. However, its essence or nature (its ontological meaning) remains unchanged, despite all the scientific, social and technological developments that have taken place. The essence of nursing is, was, and always will be, that the person (patient) must remain at the centre of all nursing interventions, actions and processes.

This relational model is still very much in its infancy in terms of conception and operation. The arrows indicate that the model is two-directional, meaning that individuals and organisations have the potential to shape, inform and influence each of the key elements – both positively and negatively. Although it could be seen as moralistic, the relational model is not actually intended to be so. Its design and development have emerged from the interpretation of empirical data and reflection upon the findings of reports on failings in care that were outlined earlier in this chapter.

The model can also be applied at three different levels – for example, at an individual/ team level (micro), organisational/institutional level (meso) or global professional/societal level (macro). We now need to briefly outline the relationship of each of the key elements numbered 1–6, and discuss how they each contribute to the overall impact and outcome of the model.

1. **Spirituality**: this is often a neglected aspect of the person and omitted from holistic care. Spirituality is uniquely defined by the individual and plays a significant part in shaping and forming the person's personal identity and sense of self in the world. The concept is intimately bound with human dignity and interaction. An individual's perceptions of spirituality may be influenced by a wide range of factors such as family, culture, education and religion.

Swinton (2006) cautions about the lack of moral and ethical boundaries associated with defining spirituality. He alerts the nursing profession to the fact that individuals have committed horrendous and heinous acts throughout human history. Swinton (2006) implies that there may be good, bad and evil aspects to some individuals' spirituality. This is a fundamental point when using the term 'spirituality' in the context of this model. Here, spirituality refers explicitly to aspects of life that are affirming and nurturing, positively validating the dignity and personhood of the individual. For nurses, this implies that all their practice must be conducted in accordance to human rights legislation and codes of professional practice. This is not to sanitise or disconnect the concept of spirituality from concepts of suffering, pain, discomfort or vulnerability that impact upon people's lives. It is simply to recognise that there are some human attitudes, values and behaviours that may be pathological, breaching laws and codes of practice and leading to violations of human dignity.

2. **Dignity**: absolute dignity is a prerequisite of humanity. It pertains to every human being and can be violated by another person but never destroyed or removed. Dignity can be shaped through social interaction and is therefore relative – as in the dignity of merit, which may be socially determined and conferred. Similarly, some aspects of dignity (such as moral stature and understanding) can change throughout life. Ultimately, dignity influences individual, team, organisational and institutional identity, and can also extend to representations of professional identity.

The elements of spirituality and dignity have been placed together to show that they are intimately connected and symbiotic in nature (represented by the broken line). Both are absolute – residing in every single human being, whether or not they are consciously aware of this (McSherry 2007). This relationship affirms that you cannot have one without the other, since both have a fundamental role in shaping and informing identity.

3. **Identity**: this word has different layers of meaning in different contexts. In this model, 'identity' refers to the characteristics displayed by an individual, organisation or profession that suggest their uniqueness and contribution, in this instance, to nursing and healthcare. These characteristics are informed, shaped and developed through a wide range of variables including societal factors and differing worldviews. Ultimately these characteristics communicate to the external world something of the individual's dignity and essence. Therefore, identity often takes the form of the public persona, revealing something of the internal disposition of the individual, organisation or profession and influencing attitudes, values and – crucially – perceptions.

4. **Attitudes**: as Chochinov (2007, p. 185) articulates very clearly, attitudes 'can be defined as an enduring, learnt predisposition to behave in a consistent way towards a given class of objects (or people), or a persistent mental or neural state of readiness to react to a certain class of objects (or people), not as they are but as they are conceived to be.' In other words, attitudes communicate our underlying values, principles and predispositions. This notion of attitudes and their impact upon behaviour is certainly a central theme in Jacobson's (2009) taxonomy. Therefore, attitudes are often predicated on aspects of life and practice that are positive or negative. The word 'enduring' implies that attitudes may persist over time. However, use of the word 'learnt' suggests that attitudes are not static but dynamic and subject to challenge, change, alteration or modification.

Change can occur as a result of education, developing understanding and insight or through what individuals experience or are exposed to, such as good leadership and role models. Running parallel to attitudes is the importance of self-awareness, introspection or reflection, as these mechanisms can aid the development, eradication or modification of poor, detrimental attitudes. Thus, positive, well-considered and developed, non-discriminatory attitudes will promote and conserve dignity, recognising the uniqueness of each individual.

5. **Approach**: it is clear that attitudes, whether held individually or collectively (as in a ward, department or profession), can have a profound impact on the approach to care and the behaviour of those providing nursing and healthcare. In this model, positive attitudes will result in good practice and high-quality care that is compassionate, dignified and respectful of the uniqueness of every person. The approach to care delivery is therefore intricately bound up with the attitudes of the individual nurse, practitioner and organisation. This is supported by Lothian and Philp (2001, p. 669), who write: 'The qualitative data cited in this article suggest that attitudes of staff greatly affect both the quality of treatment of older people and the regard given to maintaining their dignity and autonomy.'

Therefore, providing dignified and compassionate care should not be the sole responsibility of one professional group but the concern of everyone involved in the delivery of healthcare and, it could be argued, society generally. As Reid (2012, p. 218) points out, it is 'about seeing the person in the patient (the other)' and responding appropriately. Indeed, this argument could be applied to the whole of humanity – because it is about seeing the humanity within every single person, in every single interaction. It is about not being complacent and desensitised to the needs of the vulnerable or suffering human being. If the individual nurse, organisation or indeed society dismisses or fails to recognise the importance of spirituality in the context of holistic and person-centred care, this dimension will be overlooked, neglected and violated in practice. At its worst, this can lead to the objectification and dehumanisation of the person, be they patient or staff.

6. **Quality and experience of care**: the six points of this relational model collectively and sequentially demonstrate how spirituality and dignity play an important part in influencing the quality and standards of care. The model demonstrates how spirituality and dignity are interrelated and interdependent, both shaping the person's identity. The way we feel about our self therefore has a significant impact on the attitudes we display, both personally and professionally. Attitudes and values are usually well established and constant, but that does not

mean they cannot be challenged, reviewed or changed through education and exposure to positive role models. It is our attitudes that determine our behaviour and our approach to care. For example, a healthcare professional who is always pessimistic about their role and profession may be perceived negatively by patients and colleagues, thus contributing to an undesirable culture. Similarly, organisations that do not listen to patients and staff when they raise concerns about standards and quality of care may end up with a culture in which staff do not feel empowered to raise questions. By re-integrating spirituality and dignity as fundamental elements of holistic care, we can create a more humanistic and person-focused approach to care. This should enable nurses and healthcare professionals to see each person as a fellow human being in every interaction. For some patients, staff not attending to their personal, religious and spiritual beliefs may have a significant negative impact on their perception of the quality of care they are receiving.

In summary, every single nurse or healthcare professional must give careful consideration to their own personal attitudes, since attitudes shape identity and ultimately the behaviour and values of those receiving and delivering care. Organisational philosophies, values and cultures have a profound effect on the attitudes and behaviour of staff and their beliefs about what constitutes good-quality nursing and healthcare. The attitudes and expectations of those receiving nursing and healthcare are equally important. For example, patients or members of the public who are abusive, aggressive and disrespectful violate the dignity of the nurse or healthcare professional caring for them (Chochinov 2007).

At the moment the experience of some patients and their relatives falls into the categories of neglect and abuse in that it fails to acknowledge and care for the needs of the whole person. Refocusing attention on spirituality in conjunction with dignity will enable healthcare organisations to reinstate a person-centred approach to the delivery of high-quality care, counteracting the target-driven consumerist and bureaucratic agendas that have pervaded nursing and healthcare in recent times.

Conclusion

In conclusion, it is easy to get the impression that everything in the current state of nursing and healthcare (especially in the UK) is negative and bad. However, this is a grave misconception and generalisation. In my opinion, some of the major failings highlighted in recent reports can be resolved by placing the individual back at the heart of everything that we strive to do, thus refocusing on the central attribute of nursing. It is true that healthcare nowadays often appears to lose sight of the importance of people and the value of human dignity, replacing them with a cold, uncaring attitude that does not heal but brings suffering, pain and, for some people, even premature death. This is why nursing and healthcare, especially within the UK, must undertake a whole system review and continue in its drive to re-establish and safeguard the core values and principles of nursing and caring.

Patients and nurses and all those who provide care are of the utmost priority. In fact, nurses and healthcare professionals are the most precious resource any organisation possesses and should therefore be valued and their contribution acknowledged and celebrated. Spirituality and dignity are constant reminders to focus our attention on the people who are in receipt of care, rather than targets and waiting times or financial constraints, which can distract us from our primary goal. There needs to be a greater recognition and acknowledgement by society of the important contribution those in nursing and caring roles provide. Above all, there must be an open, honest and transparent culture where people can challenge and raise questions without fear of intimidation or retribution.

The relational model presented in this chapter provides a simple but profound solution to some of the problems outlined. Nursing and healthcare professionals must be more reflective, and look at the valuable contribution that concepts like spirituality and dignity make to our understanding of what it means to be human and the fundamental role these play in shaping individual and collective identity. Reviewing and applying each of the six elements described in the relational model will go some way towards changing the negative cultures that currently exist in nursing and healthcare.

Chapter summary

- Spirituality and dignity are fundamental to the delivery of holistic and person-centred care. Neglecting a person's religious, personal or spiritual beliefs may lead to a violation of their human rights and their dignity.

- The spiritual dimension of care is a constant reminder to all nurses and healthcare professionals to focus upon the person and to be compassionate and caring at all times. Failure to do this can have catastrophic consequences for those receiving and those providing care, as evidenced in several reports published in the UK.

- The relational model of care highlights the dynamic relationships and links between spirituality and dignity, and how these influence attitudes, values and behaviours that determine the culture and ultimately the quality and standards of care provided by individuals and organisations.

- Implicit in the relational model is the need for all organisations to ensure that the spirituality and dignity of those providing care is nurtured and developed, and that their contribution is acknowledged, valued and celebrated.

Suggested reading

Clarke, J. (2013). *Spiritual Care in Everyday Nursing Practice: A New Approach*. London: Palgrave Macmillan.

McSherry, W. (2006). *Making Sense of Spirituality in Nursing and Healthcare Practice: An Interactive Approach*. 2nd edn. London: Jessica Kingsley Publishers.

Swinton, J. (2006). Identity and resistance: why spiritual care needs 'enemies'. *Journal of Clinical Nursing*. **15**, 918–28.

References

Baillie, L. (2009). Patient dignity in an acute hospital setting: a case study. *International Journal of Nursing Studies*. **46**, 22–36.

Bradshaw, A. (1994). *Lighting the lamp: the spiritual dimension of nursing care*. London: Scutari Press.

Chochinov, H.M. (2007). Dignity and the essence of medicine: The A, B, C & D of dignity-conserving care. *British Medical Journal*. **335**, 184–87.

Churchill Livingstone (1996). *Churchill Livingstone's Dictionary of Nursing*. 17th edn. Edinburgh: Churchill Livingstone.

Clarke, J. (2009). A critical view of how nursing has defined spirituality. *Journal of Clinical Nursing*. **18**, 1666–73.

Clarke, J. (2013). *Spiritual Care in Everyday Nursing Practice: A New Approach*. London: Palgrave Macmillan.

Fenton, E. & Mitchell, T. (2002). Growing old with dignity: a concept analysis. *Nursing Practice*. **14**(4), 19–21.

Henderson, V. (1964). The nature of nursing. *American Journal of Nursing*. **64**, 62–68.

Howden, J.W. (1992). 'Development and Psychometric Characteristics of the Spirituality Assessment Scale'. Unpublished. PhD Dissertation. The Texas Woman's University, USA.

International Council of Nurses (2012). *Code of Ethics*.
http://www.icn.ch/who-we-are/code-of-ethics-for-nurses (accessed 4 June 2016).

International Council of Nurses (2014). *Definition of Nursing*.
http://www.icn.ch/who-we-are/icn-definition-of-nursing (accessed 4 June 2016).

Jacobson, N. (2009.) A taxonomy of dignity: a grounded theory study. *BMC International Health and Human Rights*. **9**, 3. doi:10.1186/1472-698X-9-3

Lothian, K. & Philp, I. (2001). Maintaining the dignity and autonomy of older people in the healthcare setting. *British Medical Journal*. **322** (7287), 668–70.

Males, J. & Boswell, C. (1990). Spiritual needs of people with a mental handicap. *Nursing Standard*. **4**(48), 35–37.

McSherry, W. (2006). *Making Sense of Spirituality in Nursing and Healthcare Practice an Interactive Approach*. 2nd edn. London: Jessica Kingsley Publishers.

McSherry, W. (2007). *The Meaning of Spirituality and Spiritual Care within Nursing and Healthcare Practice*. Wiltshire: Quay Books.

McSherry, W. & Smith, J. (2012). 'Spiritual Care' in W. McSherry, R. McSherry & R. Watson (eds) (2012). *Care in Nursing: Principles, Values and Skills*. Oxford: Oxford University Press.

Murray, R.B. & Zentner, J.B. (1989). *Nursing Concepts for Health Promotion*. London: Prentice Hall.

Narayanasamy, A. (2001). *Spiritual Care: a practical guide for nurses and healthcare practitioners*. 2nd edn. Wiltshire: Quay Books.

Nightingale, F. (1969.) *Notes on Nursing*. New York: Dover Publication, Inc.

Nordenfelt, L. & Edgar, A. (2005). The four notions of dignity. *Quality in Ageing*. **6**(1), 17– 21.

Pearson, A., Vaughan, B. & Fitzgerald, M. (2005). *Nursing Models for Practice*. 3rd edn. Oxford: Butterworth Heinemann.

Reed, P. (1992). An emerging paradigm for the investigation of spirituality in nursing. Research in Nursing and Health. **15**, 349–57.

Reid, J. (2012). Respect, compassion and dignity: the foundations of ethical and professional caring. *Journal of Perioperative Practice*. **22**(7), 216–19.

Royal College of Nursing (2011). *RCN spirituality survey 2010.* London: RCN.
https://www2.rcn.org.uk/__data/assets/pdf_file/0008/395864/Sprituality_online_resource_Final.pdf (accessed 4 June 2016).

Royal College of Nursing (2014). *Defining nursing.*
https://www2.rcn.org.uk/__data/assets/pdf_file/0003/604038/Defining_Nursing_Web.pdf (accessed 4 June 2016).

Stoll, R.I. (1989). 'The essence of spirituality' in V.B. Carson (ed.) *Spiritual dimensions of nursing practice.* Philadelphia: W.B. Saunders Company.

Swinton, J. (2006). Identity and resistance: why spiritual care needs 'enemies'. *Journal of Clinical Nursing.* **15**, 918–28.

Swinton, J. & Pattison, S. (2010). Moving beyond clarity: towards a thin, vague, and useful understanding of spirituality in nursing care. *Nursing Philosophy.* **11**, 226–237

Tanyi, R.A. (2002). Towards clarification of the meaning of spirituality. *Journal of Advanced Nursing.* **39**(5), 500–509.

The Mid Staffordshire NHS Foundation Trust Public Inquiry (2013). *Report of the Mid Staffordshire NHS Foundation Trust Public Inquiry.*
http://webarchive.nationalarchives.gov.uk/20150407084003/http://www.midstaffspublicinquiry.com/ (accessed 4 June 2016).

The Parliamentary and Health Service Ombudsman (2011). *Care and compassion? Report of the Health Service Ombudsman on ten investigations into NHS care of older people.* http://www.ombudsman.org.uk/__data/assets/pdf_file/0016/7216/Care-and-Compassion-PHSO-0114web.pdf (accessed 4 June 2016).

The Parliamentary and Health Service Ombudsman (2015). *Dying without dignity.*
http://www.ombudsman.org.uk/reports-and-consultations/reports/health/dying-without-dignity (accessed 4 June 2016).

The Patients Association (2009). *Patients... not numbers, People... not statistics.* Middlesex: The Patients Association.

The Patients Association (2010). *Listen to patients, Speak up for change.* Middlesex: Patients Association.

The Patients Association (2011). *We've been listening, have you been learning?* Middlesex: Patients Association.

Whitehead, J. & Wheeler, H. (2008a). Patients' experiences of privacy and dignity. Part 1: a literature review. *British Journal of Nursing.* **17**(6), 381–85.

Whitehead, J. & Wheeler, H. (2008b). Patients' experience of privacy and dignity. Part 2: an empirical study. *British Journal of Nursing.* **17**(7), 458–64.

Chapter 7

The service user and carer perspective

Lesley Baillie, Elaine Maxwell and Nicola Thomas

Introduction

There is increasing commitment to public involvement in healthcare, with healthcare providers seeking perspectives from service users (both patients and their families) – for example, through patient experience surveys, which are now well embedded in the National Health Service in the UK. Healthcare services are required to have service user involvement, with representation on NHS governing boards, service development teams and health and social care inspection teams. Gathering narratives from the patients and carers who use health services is another way of facilitating patient and carer involvement. By capturing and sharing these stories, health service providers can gain the patient and carer perspective they need in order to improve care quality. In particular, narratives can do much to illuminate human experiences of dignity in healthcare. However, it is important to consider the way in which narratives are captured and used; and we must ensure that their use is beneficial to all involved and has a positive effect on the quality of care.

In this chapter, we first set out the background to patient and public involvement in healthcare and explain associated key concepts. Next, we introduce patient and carer stories and critically review how these are being used within healthcare. A narrative from a carer's perspective is then presented, followed by an analysis using a model of dignity (Nordenfelt & Edgar 2005) and drawing on research concerning dignity in healthcare. Finally, we draw conclusions about the use of narratives in improving quality of care.

Learning objectives

This chapter will enable you to:

- Appreciate the background to patient and public involvement in healthcare and key related concepts

- Critically review the use of patient and carer stories within healthcare from a range of perspectives
- Analyse a narrative of healthcare experience in the context of a theoretical model of dignity and service user involvement
- Draw conclusions about the use of narratives in healthcare and their potential to help improve quality of care.

Background: patient and public involvement

'Patient involvement' is a complex concept and the term is sometimes used interchangeably with 'partnership' and 'participation', although these terms have a slightly different meaning. In general terms, patient involvement can be described as 'approaches which engage individual patients in the management of their health and healthcare, and in the decisions that are made in the course of it' (National Voices 2012).

A qualitative study undertaken in 15 countries in 2012 for the European Commission, found that patient involvement was not clearly understood by either patients or practitioners and often meant different things to different people (TNS Qual+ 2012). The same study found that patient involvement, in the sense of having patients at the heart of the healthcare process, seemed to be poorly understood by many professionals and patients across the EU, with very few actual ideas and activities to substantiate the concept in real healthcare practices.

Historical perspective on patient and public involvement in healthcare

During the late 1990s, there was a distinct positive shift towards patient and public involvement (PPI) in healthcare in the UK. This was partly driven by the Modernisation Agenda under the Labour Government at that time, but also because of high-profile inquiries into serious clinical and service failings – as in Bristol, England (DH 2001). The Bristol enquiry identified the need to place PPI at the centre of developing a patient safety culture. Consequently, the early 2000s saw a number of publications from the Department of Health on PPI, such as *Strengthening Accountability: Involving Patients and the Public* (2003), *A Stronger Local Voice: A Framework for Creating a Stronger Local Voice in the Development of Health and Social Care Services* (2006) and *Real Involvement: Working with People to Improve Services* (2008). It also became a legal duty in 2006 to involve patients and the public in the planning of, and changes made, to healthcare services (National Health Service Act 2006).

More recently there have been other attempts to embed PPI across NHS services in England, such as *Equity and Excellence: Liberating the NHS* (DH 2010), in which the government outlined its aspirations for an NHS that puts patients and the public first, and where 'no decision about me, without me' would become the norm. It included proposals to give everyone more say over their care and treatment, with more opportunity to make informed choices, as a way of securing better care and better outcomes. The Health and Social Care Act in 2012 clarified the duties borne by the NHS Commissioning Board and clinical commissioning groups (CCGs) to promote the involvement of patients and carers in decisions about their care and treatment, and to enable patient choice.

In summary, patient and public involvement is concerned with contributing to decisions about healthcare policy and care services, and representing the views of patients and the public, but also about individuals being involved in their own care.

Patient and public involvement programmes

Recent Care Quality Commission (CQC) patient surveys in England have shown that 48% of inpatients and 30% of outpatients want more involvement in decisions about their care (CQC 2011). It is important to note of course, that not everyone (whether patient or carer) does want to be involved in their healthcare: the extent to which involvement is desired can depend on the type and seriousness of illness, various personal characteristics and patients' relationships with particular healthcare professionals (Thompson 2007).

The Patient Participation team at NHS England are working on several programmes of work that support patients to be more actively involved in their own care, such as giving them more confidence to talk to healthcare professionals, taking steps to manage their own health and care, and helping them access and understand information to help make decisions.

These programmes of work include:

- Patient activation: patients having the right skills, knowledge and confidence to play an active role in their own care
- Patient information and health literacy
- Personalised care and support planning
- Shared decision-making and patient decision aids.

Yet, despite policy drivers to involve patients and the public, it has been argued that involvement is still not a mainstream activity that sits alongside other policy and performance requirements in the NHS (Ocloo & Fulop 2011).

Different degrees of patient and public involvement

There are many different ways in which people can participate in health, depending upon their personal circumstances and interests. The 'Ladder of Engagement and Participation'

(Arnstein 1969) is a widely recognised model for understanding different forms and degrees of patient and public involvement. Figure 7.1 (adapted from Arnstein) shows one way in which practitioners can evaluate their involvement practices, by asking themselves where on the ladder they believe their interactions with service users to be.

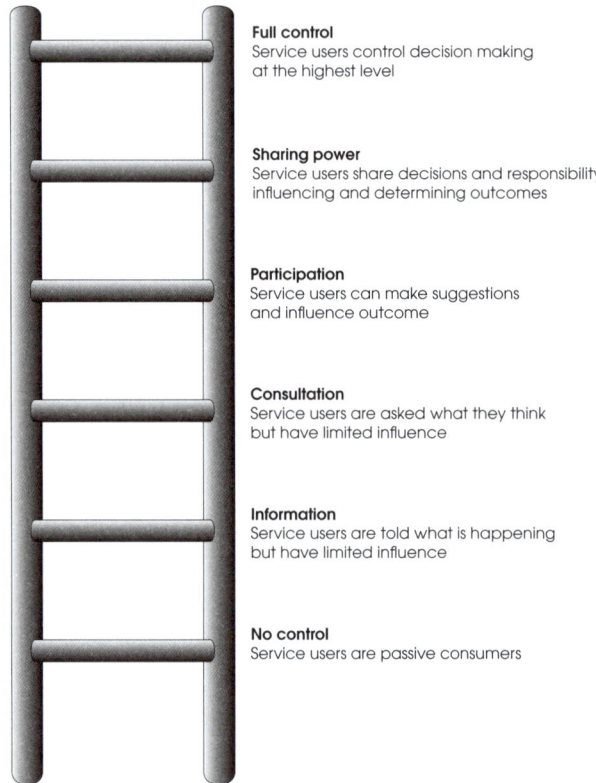

Full control
Service users control decision making at the highest level

Sharing power
Service users share decisions and responsibility, influencing and determining outcomes

Participation
Service users can make suggestions and influence outcome

Consultation
Service users are asked what they think but have limited influence

Information
Service users are told what is happening but have limited influence

No control
Service users are passive consumers

Figure 7.1 The Engagement Ladder (adapted from Arnstein 1969)

Patient and public engagement becomes increasingly valuable as the steps of the ladder are climbed, although participation becomes more meaningful at the top of the ladder. For example, there has been increasing debate about shared decision-making (sharing power) in recent years, which has been defined as a process by which 'clinicians and patients work together to select tests, treatments, management or support packages, based on clinical evidence and the patient's informed preferences' (Coulter & Collins 2011). Shared decision-making (SDM) is important for patients because of potential benefits such as improved physiological parameters through self-management programmes and increased patient satisfaction (Coulter 2009).

Use of patient and carer narratives for improving healthcare

Healthcare organisations are increasingly being encouraged to involve patients in improving care. Berwick (2013, p. 5) asserts that 'patients and their carers should be present, powerful and involved at all levels of healthcare organisations' and that they should 'advise leaders and managers by offering their expert advice on how things are going, on ways to improve, and on how systems work best to meet the needs of patients' (*ibid*, p. 20).

Barello *et al.*'s (2012) review of the literature observes that recent focus has been on engaging patients in order to manage their own physical health and suggests a lack of empirical research into the components of patient engagement at individual, relational and organisational levels. Despite this, patient stories have gained acceptance as empowerment strategy – perhaps, as Rose and Gidman (2010) contend, because stories provide an alternative form of knowledge. There is, however, little clarity about how to use their stories and they risk becoming a token response to the patient engagement agenda. One might go so far as to say it is unethical to ask a patient or relative to endure the stress of presenting their experience without a clear intended outcome.

A number of different purposes may be served by storytelling. Stories connect with people at an emotional level, and storytelling at the start of a meeting can encourage a patient-sensitive, reflective stance in subsequent discussion. Many patients, though, want their story to have a tangible, specific impact and to ensure that no one else has the same experience. Where there has been a safety failure or poor experience, patients are often frustrated by the impersonal nature of the investigations that are undertaken; they want the audience to understand the full impact of the experience on the patient, their family and friends, which goes well beyond the clinical outcome.

Organisations may have a different purpose and wish to hear patient stories at meetings as a way of helping them understand how effective their policies are in practice and how their strategic plans have influenced patients' experiences. They may also use patient stories to help set priorities in their business planning.

Whatever the reason for the telling of patient stories, it is important that they are well handled. The audience needs to understand how the storyteller has been selected. Are they considered to be representative of a group of service users or is their experience an extreme example? Is there evidence that might support their interpretation or counteract it? And does the audience need to hear any other views about the experience, particularly if there are allegations of poor conduct?

There appears to be little or no evidence about the extent to which patients and their relatives welcome the opportunity to tell their story in person and it should not be assumed that they want to share intimate experiences beyond the care team with whom they have established a relationship. Their willingness to do so may be partly influenced by the choice of media. For instance, the patient may nominate someone else to tell the story on their behalf – either an advocate or a trusted member of staff. Or they may prefer to be video or audio recorded, rather than attend a face-to-face meeting, where they might feel overwhelmed. It is important that no assumptions are made about their intentions and that several options are offered.

Given that stories can evoke strong emotions in both the teller and the listener, the session has to be well facilitated to ensure that all voices are heard and respected and to manage sensitively any criticism of individuals or organisations, in the same way as staff stories need to be well facilitated (Lown *et al.* 2010). The storyteller needs to be supported and to understand how the session will run. The audience also needs to be briefed on how their questions and comments will be handled and how to question appropriately, particularly if confidences could potentially be breached.

It is important that issues raised in the story are not left hanging at the end, and that the issues are clearly identified. The facilitator must ensure there is clarity about how these issues will be taken forward. This might mean investigating unresolved issues, or it may involve celebrating good experiences. But perhaps the most useful aspect of patient stories for service improvement is the development of questions or themes, taking the story from the concrete to the abstract, the operational to the strategic, in order to review organisational strategy and to guide quality monitoring. At Board level, it is important to search for data that is routinely collected and which can serve as an indicator of the issues raised in the story. If no data is currently available, consideration should be given to what might be collected to monitor whether the issues raised have been satisfactorily addressed.

A further step is needed in the management of patient stories: an evaluation of the session. Most importantly, there should be a chance for the storyteller to give feedback on the telling of the story. Both the storyteller and the audience might reflect on whether sufficient time was allocated to the story, especially if it is the opening item on a meeting agenda. It is also useful to reflect on how the story has been presented, and whether it might have been done differently. Finally, the story might evoke strong emotions in the audience hearing it, and it is important to ensure that there are opportunities to talk these through and provide more formal support if required.

A family carer's narrative

In this section, one of this chapter's authors, Elaine Maxwell, presents a narrative of her experience after her father was admitted to hospital following a rapid deterioration in his health. The narrative raises many issues concerning the involvement of patients and families in decision-making, and it ends with Elaine's experience of telling her story to staff at the NHS Trust and being asked if her story could be used. The narrative is analysed using Nordenfelt and Edgar's (2005) dignity model and research about dignity and illustrates how patient and carer involvement influences dignity.

'Seeing the diagnosis but not the person' written by Elaine Maxwell

My father, Delwyn, was an active man who suffered neck pain, which he put down to arthritis. At 80 he cycled around Jersey. Then, one day, he started to experience tingling in his hands. He was admitted to the local hospital and, as I had previously been Director of Nursing there, I was confident that he would be well treated.

I kept ringing the ward but they were unable to tell me anything. I eventually discovered that he had been clerked by a junior doctor but had not been reviewed by anyone senior. However, I was reassured that he was comfortable and stable and there was no need for me to come to the hospital immediately. The next day he was seen by the on-call consultant and a CT scan was performed.

When I arrived at the hospital that evening, Dad had been transferred to an orthopaedic ward and I was shocked by his condition. He was now unable to hold a cup, fasten buttons or stand. When I pointed out this deterioration, I was told that his Early Warning Score (EWS) was fine. The EWS (which is calculated using vital signs measurements) only looks at cardiac and respiratory function, and his loss of independence, mental state and a host of other functions seemed to be invisible to the team, who only seemed to be concerned with preventing cardiac arrests.

No one knew what the scan showed. I naively thought it must be OK or Radiology would have told someone but, as my father deteriorated over the weekend, I kept asking to see a doctor. No medical team doctors would come to speak to me on the orthopaedic ward and, of course, Delwyn wasn't the patient of the orthopaedic doctors. The ward sister studiously ignored me each time I went to the nurses' station to enquire.

At 5pm on the following Monday, a consultant examined my father and then asked to speak to me. The scan had shown a massive malignant spinal cord compression but he could not explain to me why this had not been discussed with a senior doctor on the Friday or why they had not put a collar on Dad or referred him to neurosurgeons. It did, however, explain why none of the junior doctors would come to see me over the weekend. The irony of sitting on a ward proudly displaying the NICE (National Institute for Health and Care Excellence) guidelines for metastatic spinal cord compression on the wall was not lost on me at this point.

The neurosurgeons were contacted and felt the tumour was too large to operate on. No one asked Delwyn or me what he would like to do but the medical team insisted on speaking to the oncologist about radiotherapy. The oncologist was keen, despite my reservations and my father's concern that it would mean being transferred to another hospital. In the meantime, I tried to get the junior medical staff to speak to my father about his resuscitation wishes. The junior doctors preferred not do so until they had the consultant's blessing but the consultant was busy; and I did wonder why they hadn't thought about these things when they were on the ward with my father themselves.

My father was transferred to another hospital and started radiotherapy, which he found extremely painful. After three days the tumour had grown significantly so it was decided that radiotherapy should stop. I will never forget the oncology registrar who told my totally paralysed father that he would have to leave, as this was an acute ward. She told him that if there were no beds in the hospice he would have to go to a community hospital 40 miles from his home but he couldn't stay in 'her' beds. Dad was distraught and in tears and it was obvious to me that he was dying and in pain. I told the nurses this but they showed me that the doctor had written in Dad's notes that he had a life expectancy of 6–9 months. (He actually died five days later.)

At this point I decided I could not leave him alone so I moved into his room to care for him myself. The Sister told me I could not stay for 'infection control' reasons; I told her she would have to get the police to remove me but I do not know how tenacious other relatives would have been in such circumstances.

Once I was resident on the ward, the nurses kept coming to tell me how busy and stressed they were, and how much pressure they were under to free up beds so that the hospital did not breach the 4-hour waiting target for emergency department admissions.

I decided not to use the official complaints procedures, as I know how demanding that is of bereaved relatives. I did write to the Chair of the NHS Trust, who asked to see me. She asked if I wanted the staff present but I did not feel able to discuss his care with them at that stage. She listened to me, then asked if I would present Delwyn's story at the Board. I told her that it was not my responsibility to manage her hospital. What I wanted to do was to pass the story to someone I trusted to act on it. I wanted to grieve for my father and not have his memory tainted by continued meetings with the hospital.

I didn't think any of the staff were bad people and I didn't want to sue them or for anyone to be sacked. I think they lacked awareness of the seriousness of Delwyn's condition and were unable to manage their own stress, let alone Delwyn's or mine.

Dad's experience illustrates the point made by Marianne Rigge, of the College of Health, in a personal communication – that the problem with evidence-based medicine is that many patients don't have evidence-based problems. Without a diagnostic label, the staff were apparently unable to understand his needs and unable to see the deterioration that was painfully obvious to me.

Critical thinking activities

1 What were the key dignity-related issues in the narrative above? Write a critical review, detailing the reasons why some of these issues might have occurred.
2 Reflect on the use of patient/carer narratives in initiatives to improve care quality: is this burdensome or empowering?
3 What lesson can you take away from Elaine's narrative about the involvement of patients and families in their care?

Analysis of Elaine's narrative

Elaine's narrative reveals the impact on her and her father of not being informed about his diagnosis in a timely or sensitive way and a lack of any involvement in decision-making, while also raising a number of dignity-related issues. In particular, there was a failure to consider Delwyn and his daughter as valued human beings who should have been involved in decisions about care. The focus on diagnosis and treatment led to Delwyn being viewed as a medical problem that could not be solved, rather than as a person who was in pain and needed care, comfort and dignity.

Nordenfelt and Edgar's (2005) theoretical model of dignity comprises four notions of dignity: *Menschenwürde*, dignity of merit, dignity of moral stature and dignity of personal identity; each of these will be further explored. As mentioned in previous chapters, *Menschenwürde* is a German word referring to the universal dignity that is inherent in all human beings and cannot be lost, reflecting the Universal Declaration of Human Rights (United Nations 1948) perspective that all human beings have equal dignity and rights. This notion of human dignity is well supported within healthcare literature, both in primary research studies based in healthcare (Matiti 2002, Jacelon 2003) and concept analyses of dignity (Jacelon *et al.* 2004, Griffin-Heslin 2005, Jacobson, 2007). This notion of universal dignity applies to each person, whatever their circumstances, and thus applies to both Delwyn and Elaine.

The other notions of dignity in Nordenfelt and Edgar's (2005) model can fluctuate between and within individuals. Dignity as merit is based on rank or status in society, either conferred at birth (as in royalty) or due to later accomplishments, and is closely linked with the original Latin word *dignitas*, which was used to describe high-ranking individuals in the Roman empire (Nordenfelt & Edgar 2005). Elaine's previous senior position in the NHS Trust implies her dignity of merit, achieved through her nursing career.

Dignity as moral stature concerns self-respect and relates to an individual's character. It concerns moral virtue and behaving according to one's own principles and values. Baillie (2009) argues that dignity of merit and dignity of moral stature have less relevance to healthcare, as nurses (and other healthcare professionals) have an ethical and professional obligation to preserve the dignity of all healthcare users. For example, healthcare professionals often care for people who would not be considered to hold dignity of moral stature within society (such as convicted sex offenders). Nevertheless, healthcare workers must recognise the human dignity of these individuals and provide care in a way that preserves that dignity.

Dignity of moral stature also relates to healthcare professionals' own behaviour. For example, raising concerns about quality of care could be considered dignity of moral stature. Staff who raise concerns are acting in accordance with their duty of care (Jackson *et al.* 2011) and maintaining the ethics of truth telling, the promotion of justice and the redressing of wrongs (Berry 2004). From a carer's perspective, Elaine's insistence about staying with Delwyn reflected her own values of doing what she believed was right for her father, portraying a dignity of moral stature. Staying with her father would have helped him to feel cared about, as a valued person, which is important for a person's dignity

(Chochinov *et al.* 2002, Jacelon 2003, Matiti 2002, Baillie 2009). Furthermore, in Slettebø *et al.*'s (2009) study, patients specifically referred to support from family and friends as a factor that preserved their dignity.

Dignity of personal identity is closely linked to a person's self-image and concerns the integrity of a person's body and mind. It is affected by the behaviour of other people, as well as changes within the person, such as illness and disability (Nordenfelt & Edgar 2005). Elaine's narrative starts by highlighting Delwyn's personal identity as a man who, at the age of 80, was still active and fit enough to be able to cycle around Jersey. The narrative illustrates how his dignity of identity was threatened by deteriorating health and how the behaviour of the hospital staff compounded the undignifying effects of his health condition. Jacobson (2007) refers to the notion of 'social dignity', which is experienced through interactions between ourselves and others and comprises two linked elements: 'dignity-of-self' (which includes self-confidence and self-respect, created through interaction); and 'dignity-in-relation' (which concerns the conveying of worth to others). In her later work, Jacobson (2009) details ways in which dignity can be violated. Almost all these violations are the result of other people's behaviour and some of them were illustrated in Elaine's narrative (as discussed below).

Elaine's recognition of her father's rapid deterioration when she visited him in the orthopaedic ward was all the more alarming because it seemed that the staff did not recognise how ill he was. They appeared to focus only on measurable aspects of Delwyn's condition, rather than focusing on him as a person. The loss of independence that Delwyn experienced, such as being unable to hold a cup or do up his buttons, should have been recognised as a significant physical deterioration that needed urgent investigation. Loss of independence has also been associated with diminished dignity (Matiti 2002, Woolhead *et al.* 2005, Baillie 2009) and would clearly affect the personal identity of an individual who had been as active as Delwyn.

Baillie (2009) found that a serious illness, or uncertainty about diagnosis, led to feelings of being out of control, which diminished dignity. In the narrative, Elaine feared that her father's diagnosis was serious and she struggled to gain information. Explanations and information-giving help people to feel in control and promote their dignity (Bayer *et al.* 2005, Enes 2003, Jacelon 2003, Matiti 2002, Baillie 2009). In addition, information is essential for patients and families if they are to make informed choices and be involved in their care and decision-making. Involvement of patients and families requires staff to be willing and able to engage with them but Elaine experienced a lack of engagement from the ward sister and the junior doctors. She described how the ward sister ignored her; both indifference and disregard (portrayed through ignoring) are behaviours that violate dignity (Jacobson 2009) as well as posing barriers to involvement in care. Elaine perceived that the junior medical staff refused to engage with her and provide information about her father's diagnosis or involve either her or Delwyn in decisions about resuscitation. The result of their lack of confidence, influenced by hospital procedures and hierarchy, led to further uncertainty for Elaine and Delwyn and a lack of involvement in important care decisions. Facilitating choice, for example in decision making, has also been found to promote dignity (Widäng & Fridlund 2003, Woolhead *et al.* 2005) but there was no evidence in the narrative of Elaine or Delwyn making any choices about care decisions.

Studies about dignity in healthcare have illuminated how the behaviour of staff affects the dignity of patients, positively or negatively (Widäng & Fridlund 2003, Baillie 2009). Baillie's (2009) research illustrated how staff behaviour can either promote or threaten the dignity of patients who are already vulnerable to indignity, due to their health conditions. The oncology registrar's words implied a focus on systems ('her' beds) with a resulting failure to see Delwyn as an individual human being, who was near the end of his life. Her stance signified a dismissal of concerns, which is a behaviour identified as a dignity violation (Jacobson 2009). Furthermore, the discussion about a move to another healthcare facility implied no involvement from either Delwyn or Elaine.

Elaine's perspective was that the staff focused on Delwyn's medical diagnosis without seeing him as an individual, and their failure to recognise and manage Delwyn's pain certainly added to his distress and hers too. The International Council of Nurses' Code of Ethics (2012) includes the statement that 'inherent in nursing is respect for human rights, including the right to life, to dignity and to be treated with respect'. However, based on the narrative, there was little regard for Delwyn's dignity, nor that of his daughter. From a legal perspective, leaving Delwyn in pain was inhumane and degrading and therefore possibly also breached the UK's Human Rights Act (Article 3).

Much of Elaine's narrative about the ward sister and nurses implies that hospital systems (including infection control policies and bed management pressures) presented barriers to caring in a way that considers the individual needs of patients and their families. Baillie's (2009) research highlighted how hospital systems threaten dignity and, in a UK-wide survey, many nurses identified hospital systems, particularly bed management, as preventing them from providing dignified care (Baillie *et al.* 2008). As Elaine recognised, the staff were not 'bad people'. However, it seemed that their priorities had become target-driven (four-hour A&E targets) and policy-bound (infection control), rather being focused on the person and family. The culture of an organisation influences the systems put in place and will affect whether staff feel supported to prioritise individual needs over organisational priorities and systems (Baillie & Black 2014).

From Elaine's viewpoint in the narrative, the Chair of the NHS Trust was concerned and interested in listening to her experience and she also offered the opportunity to speak directly to the staff and to present the experience to the Trust's Board. Elaine's response to these opportunities (that she only wanted to tell her story to the Chair at this stage) illustrates that we must make no assumptions about how patients and families may wish to share their experiences with healthcare staff. Providing choices and options gives back some control, which is an important factor influencing dignity (Matiti & Baillie 2011).

Another learning point from the narrative is that Elaine was only prepared to share her story with someone she trusted. For healthcare professionals who wish to learn from the stories of patients and families, a crucial first step is building a trusting relationship; furthermore, building relationships with patients and families promotes dignity (Baillie & Gallagher 2011). If, as in Elaine's experience, the healthcare provider has not engendered trust with the family, we must not underestimate the task of building the trust necessary for a family member to share their story. We need to recognise the exposing nature, for patients and families, of sharing personal information about themselves. Maintaining privacy of information promotes dignity (Calnan *et al.* 2005, Matiti 2002) and relates to dignity as personal identity from a personal integrity perspective. Organisations that wish to use patient and family narratives for learning purposes must therefore start with this factor in mind. It would be a travesty if the act of sharing patient or family narratives, with the intention of learning and improving care, instead led to a diminishing of dignity and a further breakdown of trust.

The narrative presented in this chapter (of the healthcare provided to an acutely unwell man and his daughter's perspective on this) has illuminated the importance of dignity and of seeing patients and their families as valued human beings. Using patient or carer narratives or stories as a basis for learning and quality improvement is one way of promoting public involvement in healthcare. However, it is important to develop trust and adopt a sensitive approach when obtaining stories from patients or carers.

Chapter summary

- Narratives can provide a more personal and holistic insight into the experiences of patients and carers than routine surveys, helping healthcare providers to contextualise experiences and appreciate service user perspectives.

- Insights from narratives have the potential to lead to quality improvement but the way in which healthcare providers gather and use narratives needs careful consideration, with a sensitive approach, clarity about their purpose and how they will be used in practice.

- Using specific patient narratives to complement quantitative data reports can be a powerful way of increasing focus and engagement with quality and safety issues.

Suggested reading

For more in-depth understanding, you are encouraged to read:

Baillie, L. (2009). Patient dignity in an acute hospital setting: a case study. *International Journal of Nursing Studies*. **46**, 22–36.

Barello, S., Graffigna, G. & Vegni, E. (2012). Patient engagement as an emerging challenge for healthcare services: mapping the literature. *Nursing Research and Practice*. **39**, 4

NHS Wales (2010). *Learning to use patient stories. 1000 Lives Plus programme*. Cardiff: NHS Wales, Cardiff. http://www.1000livesplus.wales.nhs.uk (accessed 6 June 2016).

Rose, P. & Gidman, J. (2010). 'Patient experience as evidence' in P. Rose & J. McCarthy (eds) *Values Based Health and Social Care: Beyond Evidence Based Practice*. London: Sage Publications.

References

Arnstein, S.R. (1969). A Ladder of Citizen Participation. *Journal of the American Institute of Planners*. **35**(4), 216–24

Baillie, L. (2009). Patient dignity in an acute hospital setting: a case study. *International Journal of Nursing Studies*. **46**, 22–36.

Baillie, L. & Black, S. (2014). *Professional Values in Nursing*. Taylor and Francis.

Baillie, L. & Gallagher, A. (2011). Respecting dignity in care in diverse care settings: strategies of UK nurses. *International Journal of Nursing Practice*. **17**, 336–41.

Baillie, L., Gallagher, A. & Wainwright, P. (2008). *Defending dignity: opportunities and challenges for nursing*. London: Royal College of Nursing.

Barello, S., Graffigna, G. & Vegni, E. (2012). Patient engagement as an emerging challenge for healthcare services: mapping the literature. *Nursing Research and Practice*. **39**, 4

Bayer, T., Tadd, W. & Krajcik, S. (2005). Dignity: the voice of older people. *Quality in Ageing*. **6**(1), 22–27.

Berry, B. (2004). Organizational culture: A framework and strategies for facilitating employee whistleblowing. *Employee Responsibilities and Rights Journal*. **16**(1), 1–11.

Berwick, D. (2013). *A promise to learn – a commitment to act: Improving the safety of patients in England*. London: Department of Health.

Calnan, M., Woolhead, G. & Dieppe, P. (2005). Views on dignity in providing health care for older people. *Nursing Times*. **101**(33), 38–41.

Care Quality Commission (2011). *Surveys*. http://www.cqc.org.uk/content/surveys (accessed 16 June 2016).

Chochinov, H.M., Hack, T., McClement, S., Kristjanson, L. & Harlos, M. (2002). Dignity in the terminally ill: a developing empirical model. *Social Science and Medicine*. **54**, 433–43.

Coulter, A. (2009). *Implementing shared decision making in the UK. A report for the Health Foundation*. [online] http://www.health.org.uk/sites/default/files/ImplementingSharedDecisionMakingInTheUK.pdf (accessed 16 June 2016).

Coulter, A. & Collins, A. (2011). *Making shared decision-making a reality: no decision about me, without me*. London: The King's Fund.

Coulter, A. & Ellins, J. (2007). Effectiveness of strategies for informing, educating, and involving patients. *British Medical Journal*. **335**, 24–27.

Department of Health (DH) (2001). *The Report of the Public Inquiry into Children's Heart Surgery at the Bristol Royal Infirmary 1984–1995*. London: HMSO.

Department of Health (DH) (2003). *Strengthening Accountability: Involving Patients and the Public*. London: HMSO.

Department of Health (DH) (2006). *A Stronger Local Voice: A Framework for Creating a Stronger Local Voice in the Development of Health and Social Care Services*. London: HMSO.

Department of Health (DH) (2008). *Real Involvement: Working with People to Improve Services*. London: HMSO.

Department of Health (DH) (2010). *Equity and Excellence: Liberating the NHS*. London: HMSO.

Enes, S.P.D. (2003). An exploration of dignity in palliative care. *Palliative Medicine*. **17**(3), 263–69.

Griffin-Heslin, V.L. (2005). An analysis of the concept dignity. *Accident and Emergency Nursing.* **13**(4), 251–57.

Human Rights Act (1998) c. 42. London: HMSO. http://www.legislation.gov.uk/ukpga/1998/42/contents (accessed 6 June 2016).

International Council of Nurses (2012). *The ICN Code of Ethics for Nurses.*
http://www.icn.ch/images/stories/documents/about/icncode_english.pdf (accessed 6 June 2016).

Jacelon, C.S. (2003). The dignity of elders in acute care hospital. *Qualitative Health Research.* **13** (4), 543–56.

Jacelon, C.S., Connelly, T.W., Brown, R., Proulx, K. & Vo, T. (2004). A concept analysis of dignity in older adults. *Journal of Advanced Nursing.* **48**(1), 76–83.

Jackson, D., Peters, K., Hutchinson, M., Edenborough, M., Luck, L. & Wilkes L. (2011). Exploring confidentiality in the context of nurse whistle blowing: issues for nurse managers. *Journal of Nursing Management.* **19**, 655–663.

Jacobson, N. (2007). Dignity and health: A review. *Social Science and Medicine.* **64**(2), 292–302.

Jacobson, N. (2009). Dignity violation in healthcare. *Qualitative Health Research.* **19**(11), 1536–47.

Lown, B.A. & Manning, C.F. (2010). The Schwartz Center Rounds: evaluation of an interdisciplinary approach to enhancing patient-centered communication, teamwork, and provider support. *Academic Medicine.* **85**(6), 1073–81.

Matiti, M.R. (2002). *Patient dignity in nursing: a phenomenological study.* Unpublished thesis. Huddersfield: University of Huddersfield, School of Education and Professional Development.

Matiti, M.R. & Baillie, L. (2011). 'The concept of dignity' in M.R. Matiti & L. Baillie (eds) *Dignity in Health Care for Nurses and Midwives: a practical approach for nurses and midwives.* London: Radcliffe Publishing. pp. 9–23.

National Health Service Act (2006). London: HMSO

National Health and Social Care Act (2012). London:HMSO

National Voices (2012). http://www.nationalvoices.org.uk/ (accessed 6 June 2016).

Nordenfelt, L. & Edgar, A. (2005). The four notions of dignity. *Quality in Ageing.* **6**(1), 17–21.

Ocloo, J. & Fulop, N. (2011). Developing a 'critical' approach to patient and public involvement in patient safety in the NHS: learning lessons from other parts of the public sector? *Health Expectations.* **15**, 424–32.

Rose, P. & Gidman, J. (2010). 'Patient experience as evidence' in P. Rose & J. McCarthy (eds) *Values Based Health and Social Care: Beyond Evidence Based Practice.* London: Sage Publications.

Slettebø, A., Caspari, S., Lohne, V., Aasgaard, T. & Nåden, D. (2009). Dignity in the life of people with head injuries. *Journal of Advanced Nursing.* **65**, 2426–2433.

Thompson, A. (2007) The meaning of patient involvement and participation in health care consultations: a taxonomy. *Social Science and Medicine.* **64**(6), 1297–310.

TNS Qual+ (2012). *Patient involvement aggregate report.* Brussels: European Commission.

United Nations (1948). *Universal Declaration of Human Rights.*
http://www.un.org/en/universal-declaration-human-rights/index.html (accessed 6 June 2016).

Widäng, I. & Fridlund, B. (2003). Self-respect, dignity and confidence: conceptions of integrity among male patients. *Journal of Advanced Nursing.* **42**(1), 47–56.

Woolhead, G., Calnan, M., Dieppe, P. & Tadd, W. (2005). Dignity in older age: what do older people in the United Kingdom think? *Age and Ageing.* **33**(2), 165–70.

Chapter 8

Let us not forget the dignity of the professional caregiver: the necessity of dignity preservation within the therapeutic context

Kjersti Samuelsen

Introduction

This chapter's focus is the professional relational challenges met by nurses and allied healthcare professionals, including the way therapeutic and organisational relationships may affect their personal experience of dignity. The therapeutic relationship with patients and their relatives is often described as being both rewarding and demanding. In all cases, establishing trust is of great importance. However, professional caregivers are often left alone with their own experiences, thoughts and feelings regarding caregiver interactions with patients and relatives. This chapter therefore discusses the need for self-awareness, self-caring and self-understanding, concerning dignity on both a personal and an organisational level. Lack of clinical supervision or conscious consideration of this phenomenon can affect professional caregivers' health and sense of dignity and will therefore be highlighted here.

A narrative is used to illustrate an everyday situation, portraying a dignity-challenging, nurse–patient relationship. Perspectives on dignity, developed through the research of Nora Jacobson, help establish a theoretical understanding of the narrative, illustrating the complexity of dignity.

Learning objectives

This chapter will enable you to:

● Identify relational behaviour that contributes to promotion or violation of dignity.

- Reflect on the importance of self-awareness and self-caring, and its impact on 'dignity-of-self' and 'dignity-in-relation' as a professional caregiver.
- Learn more about clinical supervision and its role as a dignity-promoting approach.

Background

Dignity is well documented as a relational and intrinsic phenomenon, contributing positively to human health – and quality of life (Chochinov *et al.* 2002; Valentine, Darby & Bonsel 2008). Although healthcare professionals are often looked upon as having high social status, preserving their own dignity is a subject that is poorly investigated and should be of growing concern (Lawless & Moss 2007, Berg & Danielson 2007). In this chapter, the experience of dignity in therapeutic relationships, especially from the caregiver's perspective, will be emphasised. This chapter will mainly focus on the need for clinical supervision, and how growing awareness on both the individual and relational level may contribute to a broader understanding of the complex concept of dignity. This text also acknowledges how theoretical perspectives on dignity as a human phenomenon can contribute to this understanding.

Through searches in the databases CINAHL, PubMed, Embase and PsycINFO, it is recognised that dignity is closely related to other subjects, such as work–life environment, organisational culture, stress and burnout. It is clear that these subjects are intertwined, and this may also contribute to the discussion of what the phenomenon of dignity really entails.

There have been very few studies investigating nurses and allied healthcare professionals' dignity, and the effect of clinical supervision on their dignity experience. Some of the research presented below, conducted by Gallagher (2004), Lawless and Moss (2007), Sabatino *et al.* (2014), Stievano *et al.* (2013), Khademi, Mohammadi and Vanaki (2012), use the word 'dignity' explicitly in their investigations and conclusions, thus strengthening their relevance to this discussion.

Other researchers, like Faulkner and Laschinger (2008), Honkavuo and Lindström (2014), and Bridges *et al.* (2012), do not specifically direct their attention to dignity in their work. However, empowerment and courtesy are, in the work of Nora Jacobson (2009), recognised as dignity-promoting elements, which are also crucial to the concepts of respect and support: 'Respect, on the other hand, is not the same thing as dignity, but is a property of the external social processes that may promote it' (Jacobson & Silva 2010, p. 367). These studies are therefore valuable within this present discussion.

Through the theoretical lens of Nora Jacobson (2007, 2009, 2010, 2012), issues relating to recognition, empowerment, acceptance and love are documented as being crucial for people's dignity. These concepts are used as a theoretical framework for discussing clinical supervision and its contribution to dignity promotion, which can potentially strengthen dignity among professional caregivers. This discussion will be presented later in the chapter. Although the concept of dignity is frequently mentioned in nursing literature and professional codes of nursing practice, it is almost always seen from the patient's perspective (Lawless & Moss 2007). Over the years, nursing practice and literature have embedded dignity as a core value, particularly the 'dignity of others'. In contrast, the dignity of nurses (both as a concept, and as a right of all workers and human beings) has received little explicit attention. However, there seems to be growing interest in this field, and some of the findings will be presented here. Sabatino *et al.* (2014, p. 9) suggest the following definition for 'nursing professional dignity':

> A multidimensional intertwined concept composed of the characteristics of human beings: intrinsic human dignity, subjective perception of one's own dignity, the professional identity of nurses, and their ethical values and workplace elements, including inter- and intra-professional relationships, communications with patients and their significant others, and the organizational characteristics of work environments…

These findings match those of other investigations showing how directing attention towards nurse dignity may not only benefit nurses and increase their sense of satisfaction, but also benefit their patients and organisations (Lawless & Moss 2007, Stievano *et al.* 2013). Gallagher (2004) states in her article on dignity in nursing practice, that dignity should be seen as a two-pronged professional value: as an other-regarding value and as a self-directed value, where respect for one's own (nurse's) dignity is given less attention. Lawless and Moss (2007) also raise the question: do nurses have intrinsic value as *persons* in the world, and do they deserve dignity?

In a study from Iran, nurses reported dignity violation in the form of irreverence, coercion and violation of autonomy, ignorance of their scientific and professional ability, and denial of the value of nursing and caring in the process of medical care. Here, patients and their families, physicians, structure, the principles of their governing system, and, particularly, the nursing managers were vital influencing factors (Khademi, Mohammadi & Vanaki 2012). Nursing managers are also considered as important contributors to dignity-related issues in research conducted by Faulkner and Laschinger (2008). This study documents how hospital nurses who perceive themselves as being structurally and psychologically empowered are more likely to feel respected in their workplace. Nursing managers have the influence and resources to facilitate empowering work conditions, thus enhancing nurses' feelings of being respected. The study also stresses the need to promote collaborative, inter-professional and intra-professional relationships, while ensuring continuous support for each nurse, as important strategies to build respect.

The issue of support is also addressed through leadership and clinical supervision. Nursing managers have a responsibility to offer each nurse a nursing communion (meaning a work environment that all perceive as safe, confidential and meaningful, and in which relational interactions are founded upon respect and trust). Hidden suffering among nurses, who bear the burden of confidentiality, can give rise to feelings of deep loneliness. As documented by Honkavuo and Lindstrøm (2014), such suffering may be alleviated through conversations and professional relationships between nurses and their managers. Bridges *et al.* (2012) underscore the need to establish caring cultures that more visibly value and support therapeutic relationships across organisations, reflecting the emotional needs of all parties involved. Ensuring that clinical supervision and peer support are routinely available and accessible to the entire nursing staff is also regarded as crucial.

Entering the therapeutic relationship is an everyday act for nurses and other healthcare professionals. In their study on caring relationships between nurses and patients, Berg and Danielson (2007) describe nurses' experience of the therapeutic relationship as demanding and rewarding at the same time. This chapter will discuss how clinical supervision can affect nurses and allied healthcare professionals in their work. By enhancing their self-awareness and their understanding of the therapeutic relationship, professional caregivers can increase their personal insight into the way dignity evolves within a working relationship, including learning to understand their personal reactions and feelings. This can potentially improve their practice skills – in terms of taking care of themselves as well as protecting their own 'dignity-of-self'. This chapter mainly focuses on findings related to the area of nursing, but may be transferable to other professional caregiving contexts.

Nurse Sarah's story

In the following narrative, Sarah (an experienced nurse) is working in an intensive care unit with a patient who she gradually finds challenging to relate to. This narrative has been chosen to illustrate the complexity and variety of therapeutic relationships that nurses and other healthcare professionals may become involved in.

Defending my dignity – being professional, but still vulnerable

One evening shift my colleague informed me I was to receive a new patient. Mrs Johnson was a woman with chronic obstructive pulmonary disease, and her arterial blood gas examination attested to severe CO_2-retention and lack of oxygen. This made it difficult for her to breathe normally, leading to exhaustion and anxiousness. Her ventilation therefore needed to be supported by a BIPAP (biphasic positive airway pressure) machine to normalise her blood gas status. The patient appeared otherwise to be a well-organised, mentally healthy woman. When Mrs Johnson arrived, I introduced myself to her and tried to explain why she needed a tight mask over her face. She agreed to the treatment and I placed the mask on and arranged her pillows for her. I also gave Mrs Johnson an alarm bell and showed her how she should use it to call for help.

Approximately 30 minutes later, Mrs Johnson used the alarm to ask for a cup of coffee and something to eat. She also wanted to make a phone call and use the toilet. I explained how important her treatment was, requesting she kept her mask on while using the toilet-chair I placed next to her bed. I then went out to find her some food and drink. When I returned to Mrs Johnson she had taken off her mask and was clearly angry about her present situation. She refused to place the mask back on her face, and I re-examined her blood gas, checking her status once again. Since her arterial catheter was not functioning well, I went to find a colleague to help. At this point, Mrs Johnson became even more annoyed, requesting that I improve my language skills, and find a native nurse who could speak her language properly. When the second nurse entered the room, Mrs Johnson ignored me, giving thanks and appreciation to my colleague instead. Complaining about the care I had given her, she referred to me as if I were not present.

The rest of that evening, Mrs Johnson's eyes never met mine. When I spoke to her, she rolled her eyes or acted in a somewhat childish way. At one point, I said to her: 'Excuse me, but I find it extremely difficult to help you. It would seem you are not at all interested in following my instructions, and honestly, I find your behaviour towards me quite disrespectful.' Afterwards, she merely stared at me, then turned her attention back to the television. Even though I felt exhausted and tired due to her behaviour towards me, I continued answering Mrs Johnson's alarm calls. I assumed she had difficulties that might explain her behaviour. Despite the fact that I experienced being her caregiver as unpleasant, I wanted to show her I was not afraid of her. I also wanted to demonstrate my professionalism, be polite, give her correct medical treatment, and assure her of my willingness to assist her. I think my desire was to show Mrs Johnson care and respect, even though she would not show the same in return.

Critical thinking activities

1 How do you evaluate Sarah's actions towards Mrs Johnson?

2 Reflect on your own experiences of dignity. Describe one situation when your dignity was promoted and one where it was violated. What social processes were involved? What were the contextual conditions (i.e. the positions, relationship, setting and social order)?

3 How do you think professional caregivers can enhance their ability to care for their own dignity in therapeutic relationships?

Discussion

'Dignity exists in a state of some peril. It can be "taken away"' Nora Jacobson (2012, p. 1).

Understanding Nurse Sarah's story, using Nora Jacobson's perspectives on dignity

As we learned from the description of Nora Jacobson's taxonomy in Chapter 1 of this book, two distinct forms of dignity have been documented: human dignity and social dignity (Jacobson 2007, 2009a). Social dignity can be divided into dignity-of-self and dignity-in-relation. Utilising these two perspectives, Sarah's experience of dignity can be interpreted on two levels: firstly, as having a *self* and being independent of the influence of others; and secondly, as having a form of dignity that is dependent on and influenced by being *in relation* to others. In other words, Sarah has an intrinsic dignity, just by being human, while, at the same time, she is vulnerable to the experience of having her dignity violated in her relational interactions. The therapeutic relationship may be viewed as the cornerstone of professional nursing practice, and can be defined as 'a professional, interpersonal alliance in which the nurse and client join together for a defined period to achieve health-related treatment goals' (Arnold, 2011, p. 81). It is important to acknowledge that the relationship is not necessarily voluntary, and it is by nature asymmetrical, although interdependency may be viewed as an ideal (*ibid.*).

Sarah's interaction with Mrs Johnson reveals several social processes that are dignity violating (Jacobson 2009); Mrs Johnson offends Sarah's ethnicity when she tells her to improve her language and find a nurse that shares Mrs Johnson's nationality. She also questions Sarah's value and position as a nurse when ignoring Sarah in front of her colleague. This can be perceived to correspond with what Jacobson (2009) refers to as 'rudeness' (i.e. making hurtful comments or showing general disrespect). It can also be interpreted as 'discrimination' (i.e. treating someone badly, based on their status or apparent membership of a low-status group). Furthermore, Mrs Johnson shows 'indifference', not taking Sarah's advice to keep her mask on seriously. Mrs Johnson continues to show indifference by demanding that Sarah finds another nurse, without considering Sarah's vulnerability or respecting her value. When Sarah's colleague is present, Mrs Johnson ignores her, again demonstrating a lack of respect for a competent nurse professional, something Jacobson (2009) refers to as 'diminishment' or 'disregard'. This is also demonstrated when Mrs Johnson evaluates the second nurse as being more 'important', showing more willingness to follow the second nurse's instructions, and giving *her* all the appreciation in spite of Sarah's competent efforts.

Obviously, Mrs Johnson is the more vulnerable partner in this relationship, yet she becomes the most dominant, which makes this therapeutic relationship very interesting. According to Jacobson (2009), dignity violations are more likely to occur when one part of a relationship is in a state of 'vulnerability' (i.e. being sick, poor, helpless or confused). One can therefore raise the question: who is the vulnerable partner in this relationship – Sarah or Mrs Johnson? It might be appropriate to say that they are *both* vulnerable – and dependent upon one another to make their relationship work in a dignity-preserving manner. For Sarah it becomes difficult when Mrs Johnson refuses to cooperate in numerous ways; and Mrs Johnson, from her position, might find it equally difficult to connect with Sarah.

Jacobson (2009) argues that dignity violation is connected to the behaviour of the other partner in a relationship, and this is also known as a 'position of antipathy'. This means that Mrs Johnson may perceive Sarah as being prejudiced, arrogant, hostile or impatient, and/or that Sarah may have similar feelings regarding Mrs Johnson. While Sarah may feel that she is helping Mrs Johnson in the best possible way, Mrs Johnson may perceive Sarah's care as extremely difficult to put up with, or even dignity violating. This perception may be connected to an earlier trauma, or due to Mrs Johnson's difficulties in being dependent on, or trusting another person. In addition, Mrs Johnson may see herself as someone who normally has more power and authority than someone like Sarah. Alternatively, Mrs Johnson's behaviour can be interpreted as a 'projection', expressing feelings of contempt towards her own dependency or weakness.

In Sarah's case, it is easy to understand why she feels the need to protect herself as she experiences Mrs Johnson's behaviour as rude and discriminating. If such feelings also affect Sarah's behaviour negatively, they could paradoxically 'confirm' Mrs Johnson's projection that Sarah cannot be trusted. One can also understand Mrs Johnson's behaviour as an effort to counteract an experience of asymmetry: being sick of course makes her feel more vulnerable because it forces her to give up some of her control and autonomy in life. According to Jacobson (2007, 2009), dignity violation is more likely to occur whenever a relationship is influenced by 'asymmetry' (i.e. one of the partners has more power, more authority, knowledge, strength or wealth than the other). However, it is also worth bearing in mind that a therapeutic relationship is by its nature asymmetric – one partner always being dependent upon the other's knowledge or skills. While being a professional caregiver, on whom Mrs Johnson is dependent, it becomes challenging for Sarah to balance this asymmetry. Therefore, Sarah attempts to demonstrate her willingness to balance the asymmetry in other ways. Her dignity-promoting efforts and actions will be discussed later in this chapter.

In Sarah's interaction with Mrs Johnson it may be appropriate to say there is a lack of confidence between them. Jacobson (2009) underscores the fact that dignity is promoted when one of the partners in an encounter is in a 'position of confidence' (i.e. having a sense of hope, self-assurance and feeling that they deserve good things to happen). However, this often depends on the other person's 'position of compassion', which can be interpreted as human qualities such as kindness, open-mindedness, while carrying the best intentions. In this present relationship, however, it becomes difficult for Sarah to be compassionate with her patient, since Mrs Johnson expresses her mistrust towards her, while at the same time violating Sarah's 'social dignity' in the presence of others. This makes it hard for them to establish a relationship characterised by 'solidarity', which is based on qualities like reciprocity, empathy and trust.

It is also important to consider the social setting where this encounter takes place. Professional caregivers working in a hospital setting do not always reflect on how dependency can affect the patient–caregiver relationship, but it should be remembered that being in need of care may be challenging for their patients' self-respect as well as their dignity. Jacobson (2009) describes how social settings can contribute to the promotion or violation of dignity, and explains that settings can be characterised by 'harsh circumstances' (such as being hierarchical, rigid, full of stress, distractions or lacking in resources). The dignity violation here is connected to an 'order of inequality', a social order where different forms of inequity are common. Applying this to the story of Sarah and Mrs Johnson, one may wonder if Mrs Johnson's behaviour is partly a reaction to these circumstances. In any emergency ward, the staff often need to act in an efficient manner while performing intimate procedures. For instance, removing a patient's clothing and inserting a urine catheter is an everyday act for healthcare professionals, and they often have little time to establish a relationship with their patient. It is therefore essential for professional caregivers to consider their work environment from their patient's perspective, and reflect on how they can make the setting more inclusive, building trust and security for the patient. Jacobson's research (2012) suggests that more attention should be given to aesthetics and the egalitarian use of space.

Although Sarah's interaction with Mrs Johnson contains several examples of dignity violation, it is also worth reflecting upon the ways in which Sarah tries to *promote* dignity in their relationship. According to Jacobson (2009, 2010), several processes are recognised as contributing towards the promotion of dignity. In many ways, one may say being a nurse is in itself a contributing factor because nurses 'give something' to others. By using one's personality, talents and professional competence, one gives someone else the opportunity to enhance their health status and improve their life situation. Sarah also shows the ability to 'hold back' her frustration and act in a polite manner towards Mrs Johnson, never losing her temper. Jacobson (2009) refers to this as 'restraint' but it could also be interpreted as 'concealment', where one covers up what easily could have been perceived as embarrassing behaviour.

Sarah also shows Mrs Johnson that she is willing to be 'present' for her in her difficult circumstances, meeting her nourishment and toilet needs. By introducing herself to Mrs Johnson, giving her information on how she can call upon her for help (showing her the alarm bell and answering it), Sarah demonstrates 'courtesy'. One may also argue that Sarah demonstrates her 'dignity-of-self', when confronting Mrs Johnson concerning her behaviour. Sarah is courageous when she shows Mrs Johnson she is not afraid of her, remaining both strong and present, despite the fact that she feels Mrs Johnson's disrespect. All in all, Sarah's actions contribute towards promoting 'dignity-in-relation'. One can also see the connection between Sarah's dignity-of-self and dignity-in-relation, showing how the two forms of social dignity intertwine, each bilaterally affecting the other, and one possibly promoting and strengthening the other.

Clinical supervision: promoting dignity among professional caregivers

Investigations documenting how clinical supervision enhances nurses or other allied healthcare professionals' ability to preserve dignity-of-self and dignity-in-relation are few, although it has been claimed that such supervision may help maintain personal integrity (De Raeve 1998). It is, however, acknowledged that dignity is one of the core ethical issues in clinical supervision (Berggren, da Silva & Severinsson 2005). Despite this lack of empirical evidence, one can argue that Nora Jacobson's (2009, 2010, 2012) perspectives on dignity are relevant in this context. According to Jacobson and Silva (2010, p. 367), promoting dignity is described 'as a deliberate attitude, behavior, or action engaged by an identifiable actor with the aim of creating, maintaining, defending or reclaiming dignity'. Dignity promotion may also be the byproduct or indirect consequence of an individual's attitude, behaviour or action. When aiming to promote dignity-in-relation in the act of professional caregiving, qualities such as courtesy, recognition, acceptance, generosity, presence, love, advocacy, levelling and empowerment are emphasised (Jacobson & Silva 2010, Jacobson 2012). Through such attitudes and subsequent actions, the caregiver can also promote their dignity-of-self (*ibid.*).

The concept of clinical supervision (CS) is frequently mentioned in nursing and professional caring practice, but it is not easily defined. This is an important issue when discussing CS, since uncertainty concerning its mandate may cause resistance among professional caregivers. It may also affect their motivation and willingness to participate (Cutcliffe & Proctor 1998). As the nursing profession has a great variety of practice settings, a clear definition cannot easily be formulated. However, in his concept analysis, Lyth (2000, p. 728) proposes the following definition:

> Clinical supervision is a support mechanism for practicing professionals within which they can share clinical, organizational, developmental and emotional experiences with another professional in a secure, confidential environment in order to enhance knowledge and skills. This process will lead to an increased awareness of other concepts including accountability and reflective practice...

CS is, first and foremost, focused on the recipient of the supervision – that is, the professional practitioner. The supervisor is responsible for creating a climate and a relationship in which the practitioner can reflect on their practice, with clear limits of freedom and responsibility (Proctor 2011). This CS relationship is founded upon ethical guidelines and professional codes; and, importantly, the relationship becomes in many ways a *therapeutic* one. The supervisee may experience being the vulnerable partner, making the CS relationship a reflection of the caregiver–patient relationship (Holm Wiebe *et al.* 2011). The issue of trust and asymmetry will be introduced, giving the professional practitioner the opportunity to experience these crucial relational aspects in a *personal* way (Proctor 2011). During CS, it is important to acknowledge that changes in consciousness, insight and relational behaviour can give rise to uncomfortable feelings, affecting one's own experience of self. Acknowledging previously unconscious shortcomings can be painful. Being given an opportunity to participate in reflective dialogue therefore allows one to focus on individual free choice, hopefully leading to a discovery of the benefits of CS (*ibid.*). This approach can be utilised to stimulate self-awareness and as a tool to help develop personal and professional resources concerning dignity promotion. Supporting the professional caregiving practitioner in viewing their therapeutic relationships in a more reflective manner may lead to increasing opportunities for new and broader discoveries, also allowing for the possibility of a more conscious way of 'being-in-relation'.

In the following section, the themes of recognition, empowerment, acceptance and love within CS will be more closely examined. Relevant studies will be applied in order to strengthen their connection to dignity promotion. These themes may be viewed as participating factors that give professional caregivers an opportunity to strengthen their dignity-of-self, while simultaneously enhancing their own skills in establishing and maintaining dignity-in-relation, within their therapeutic relationships.

Being recognised, and learning to recognise oneself

Recognition can be defined as 'the acknowledgement of something as valid or as entitled to consideration' or as 'acknowledgement of the right to be heard or given attention' (*Webster's Encyclopedic Unabridged Dictionary of the English Language* 1996, p. 1199). Bégat and Severinsson (2006) found that one effect of CS was the emergence and growth of self-recognition. The effect becomes evident when the professional practitioner realises and understands how taking part in CS has a positive influence on their existence and well-being. The emergence of self-recognition relates to the simultaneous discovery of themselves, as professionals and as authentic human beings. CS also provides an avenue for professional caregivers to demonstrate active support for one another. Through sharing and understanding, one can recognise the fact that one is 'not alone', and that one in fact shares similar feelings and perceptions with others. This provides reassurance and validation for personal experience and individual perceptions (Brunero & Stein-Pabury 2008).

Experiencing empowerment and acceptance – leading to authenticity and integration

Berggren and Severinsson (2000) argue that nurses who have participated in CS have gained increased self-assurance and become better able to develop authentic relationships with their patients. These nurses also developed their capacity to assume greater responsibility and act accordingly. In ethically challenging caring situations, CS proved helpful for the supervisee. CS helped increase nurses' ability to reflect on core human concerns, thereby strengthening their professional identity (Berggren, da Silva & Severinsson 2005). Experiencing shortcomings due to an inability to encounter patients or establish a good relationship may give rise to feelings of suffering. Negative feelings, such as anger, injustice, self-pity or powerlessness, may affect supervisees in a way that leads to feeling disheartened and insecure. This can damage their self-confidence and ability to trust others (Holm Wiebe *et al.* 2011). Experiencing inadequacy is common in caring situations, and this feeling is also associated with burnout. In a nursing supervision context, the supervisees' experiences of weakness is not concealed, but rather accepted, then given space to exist. It is of great importance to acknowledge and accept oneself as being weak, and at the same time a strong and competent professional (*ibid.*).

Acceptance is also linked to the ability to contain other people's feelings. Containing patients' feelings demands a nurse with an understanding of the patients' characters and how they normally respond in different situations, as these aspects are connected to self-awareness and self-acceptance. When a nurse is able to contain their patients' emotions, it is likely that the patient will feel comforted and accepted as they are (Bégat & Severinsson 2001).

Receiving love through confirmation

Receiving confirmation is the most valuable component for achieving professional growth. Confirmation is connected to the deepest human need and desire, the need to feel loved and approved of (Holm Wiebe *et al.* 2011). Confirmation includes accepting supervisees, while enabling them to gain additional insight through new discoveries (Severinsson 2001). Not being confirmed means not being seen fully or taken seriously, something which may affect a person's sense of dignity (Nåden & Eriksson 2000). Confirmation may also be seen as a tool that helps exclude doubt about experiences of reality, thus contributing to one's sense of identity (Severinsson 2001).

Receiving supervision may also be interpreted as a confirmation in itself – expressing the fact that one is needed as a human being and as a professional practitioner (Holm Wiebe *et al.* 2011). According to Severinsson (1995), a theoretical approach to caring in CS should also include a spiritual dimension, since supervision may offer an opportunity to adopt a more merciful and forgiving attitude towards oneself. Relief of guilt, understanding of one's own behaviour and experience of forgiveness and reconciliation can give the professional practitioner a stronger competency in building trust and counteracting feelings of loneliness. If a foundation of hope and faith can be established, the professional caregiver may develop and maintain a feeling of 'love' towards other people (*ibid.*).

Potential benefits for Sarah and her patient Mrs Johnson

When describing a narrative, it is never possible to portray the situation in a totally 'objective' manner, since there will always be a range of different subjective interpretations of the same series of events. For instance, in Sarah and Mrs Johnson's interaction, one might ask why their attempt to establish a positive and trustful relationship apparently failed? Did Sarah invest enough time in laying the foundations for a meaningful relationship with Mrs Johnson? Was her approach anchored in attitudes and behaviour that promoted dignity-in-relation or dignity-of-self in her and Mrs Johnson? Was Mrs Johnson never interested in a relationship with Sarah? Was she simply rejecting her?

In a CS context, a core question is not how to proceed, but rather how to be a sensitive, listening and supportive human being with professional knowledge (Severinsson 2001). For Sarah, receiving CS might not give her 'quick and simple' answers as to *why* she failed in her interactions with Mrs Johnson. Rather, it could help create an opportunity to make new discoveries, allowing her to experience and develop increased consciousness and 'self-awareness' concerning her way of being. Allowing Sarah to express her feelings would give her the ability to experience 'recognition' and 'acceptance'. Giving her the possibility of gaining new personal and professional insight may also be 'empowering' and is likely to strengthen her sense of identity. Most importantly, CS could contribute towards 'confirming' her value both as a human being and as a professional caregiver. One could then imagine that it would be easier for Sarah to encounter Mrs Johnson a second time, making new efforts (this time in a more reflective manner) and maybe even making new discoveries in their interactions with each other.

The work of Nora Jacobson (2012) acknowledges the fact that some clients are harder to treat with dignity than others. Patients who 'sabotage' their own treatment by ignoring advice, breaking agreements or not showing up, or who guard their rights so zealously that they put their care providers on the defensive, can also make it hard for professional caregivers to promote dignity-in-relation. In fact, this kind of behaviour is often a response to previous dignity violations, and can make such clients vulnerable to similar experiences that only confirm their past negative interactions.

Gallagher (2004) states that dignity should be considered as a two-pronged professional value. This includes the need for healthcare professionals to understand dignity in a fuller sense, not only from an objective point of view – as a basis for human rights. They must understand it for *themselves*, subjectively, discovering and taking on board individual differences and idiosyncrasies. When experiencing respect for their own dignity-of-self, each individual may develop their ability to envision the needs of others while finding ways to establish more respectful attitudes and behaviour (Gallagher 2004, Jacobson 2012).

Healthcare professionals encounter certain expectations in their work. For instance, patients may project previous painful, dignity-violating experiences on to current therapeutic relationships. It is therefore important to assist professional caregivers in their work, offering them strategies to discover themselves and other ways of being. The physical care environment and lack of resources should also be taken into account (Baillie & Gallagher 2012). Today, there is increasing evidence documenting the potential benefits of CS – how it can positively affect the lives of professional caregivers and, in turn, those they care for. As nurses are expected to take on ever greater responsibility for vulnerable human beings, an appropriate support network (encouraging exploration of personal and professional attitudes and behaviour) can offer increasing benefit (Lyth 2000) when aiming to enhance dignity-in-relation, as well as dignity-of-self, among all those involved in therapeutic relations.

Chapter summary

- The therapeutic relationship differs from other relationships, with its client-centred focus. Health professionals will therefore meet other needs and expectations in their work, and there is a need for awareness and competence regarding how best to promote dignity-in-relations.

- Clinical supervision can support health professionals, helping them develop self-awareness, relieving difficult emotions in a safe environment, and preventing burnout, while developing valuable personal experiences concerning vulnerability and dignity.

- Experiencing empowerment, recognition, love and acceptance in clinical supervision can contribute towards empowering professional caregivers to strengthen their dignity-of-self as well as their competence in establishing and maintaining dignity-in-relation.

Suggested reading

For more in-depth understanding, you are encouraged to read:

Cutcliffe, J.R., Hyrkäs, K. & Fowler, J. (2011). *Routledge Handbook of Clinical Supervision. Fundamental international themes.* USA/Canada: Routledge.

Jacobson, N. (2012). *Dignity & Health.* Nashville: Vanderbilt University Press.

Todaro-Franceschi, V. (2013). *Compassion fatigue and burnout in nursing. Enhancing professional quality of life.* New York: Springer Publishing Company.

References

Arnold, E.C. (2011). 'The nurse-client relationship' in E.C. Arnold & K.U. Boggs (2011). *Interpersonal relationships. Professional communication skills for nurses.* 6th edn. USA: Elsevier Saunders. pp. 83–102.

Baillie, L. & Gallagher, A. (2012). Raising awareness of patient dignity. *Nursing Standard.* **27**(5), 44–49.

Bégat, I. & Severinsson, E.I. (2001). Nurses' reflections on episodes occurring their provision of care – an interview study. *International Journal of Nursing Studies.* **38**, 71–77.

Bégat, I. & Severinsson, E.I. (2006). Reflection on how clinical supervision enhances nurses' experiences of well-being related to their psychosocial work environment. *Journal of Nursing Management.* **14**, 610–16.

Berg, L. & Danielson, E.I. (2007). Patients' and nurses' experiences of the caring relationship in hospital: an aware striving for trust. *Scandinavian Journal of Caring Sciences.* **21**, 500–506.

Berggren, I. & Severinsson, E.I. (2000). The influence of clinical supervision on nurses' moral decision-making. *Nursing Ethics.* **7**(2), 124–33.

Berggren, I., da Silva, A.B. & Severinsson, E.I. (2005). Core ethical issues of clinical supervision. *Nursing and Health Sciences.* **7**, 21–28.

Bridges, J., Nicholson, C., Maben, J., Pope, C., Flatley M., Wilkinson C., Meyer, J. & Tziggili, M. (2012). Capacity for care: meta-ethnography of acute nurses' experiences of the nurse-patient relationship. *Journal of Advanced Nursing.* **69**(4), 760–72.

Brunero, S. & Stein-Parbury, J. (2008). The effectiveness of clinical supervision in nursing: an evidenced based literature review. *Australian Journal of Advanced Nursing.* **25**(3), 86–94.

Chochinov, H.M., Hack, T., Hassard, T., Kristjanson, L.J., McClement, S. & Harlos, M. (2002). Dignity in terminally ill: A cross-sectional, cohort study. *The Lancet.* **21/28**(360), 2026–30.

Cutcliffe, J.R., Hyrkäs, K. & Fowler, J. (2011). *Routledge Handbook of Clinical Supervision. Fundamental international themes.* USA/Canada: Routledge.

Cutcliffe, J.R. & Proctor, B. (1998). An alternative training approach to clinical supervision. *British Journal of Nursing.* **7**(5), 280–85.

De Raeve, L. (1998). Maintaining integrity through clinical supervision. *Nursing Ethics.* **5**, 486–96.

Faulkner, J. & Laschinger, H. (2008). The effects of structural and psychological empowerment on perceived respect in acute care nurses. *Journal of Nursing Management.* **16**(2), 214–21.

Gallagher, A. (2004). Dignity and respect for dignity – two key health professional values: implications for nursing practice. *Nursing Ethics.* **11**(6), 587–99.

Holm Wiebe, A.-K., Johansson, I., Lindquist, I. & Severinsson, E. (2011). 'Nurses' experience of core phenomena in the supervisor training programme' in J.R. Cutcliffe, K. Hyrkäs & J. Fowler (eds) *Routledge Handbook of Clinical Supervision. Fundamental international themes.* USA/Canada: Routledge. pp.241–49.

Honkavuo, L. & Lindström, U. (2014). Nurse leaders' responsibilities in supporting nurses experiencing difficult situations in clinical nursing. *Journal of Nursing Management.* **22**, 117–26.

Hyrkäs, K., Appelqvist-Schmidlechner, K. & Lemponen R. (2011). 'Efficacy of clinical supervision. Influence on job satisfaction, burnout and quality of care' in J.R. Cutcliffe, K. Hyrkäs & J. Fowler (eds) *Routledge Handbook of Clinical Supervision. Fundamental international themes*. USA/Canada, Routledge. pp. 250–60.

International Council of Nurses (ICN) (2011). *The ICN Code of Ethics for Nurses*. Geneva: ICN.

Jacobson, N. (2007). *Dignity and health: A review. Social Science & Medicine*. **64**, 292–302.

Jacobson, N. (2009a). A taxonomy of dignity: a grounded theory study. *BMC International Health and Human Rights*. **9**: 3. doi: 10.1186/1472-698X-9-3.

Jacobson, N. (2009b). Dignity Violation in Health Care. *Qualitative Health Research*. **19**(11), 1536–47.

Jacobson, N. (2012). *Dignity & Health*. Nashville: Vanderbilt University Press.

Jacobson, N. & Silva, D.S. (2010). Dignity Promotion and Beneficence. *Bioethical Inquiry*. **7**, 365–72.

Khademi, M., Mohammadi, E. & Vanaki, Z. (2012). Nurses' experiences of violation of their dignity. *Nursing Ethics*. **19**(3), 328–40.

Lawless, J. & Moss, C. (2007). Exploring the value of dignity in the work-life of nurses. *Contemporary Nurse: a Journal for the Australian Nursing Profession*. **24**, 225–36.

Lyth, G.M. (2000). Clinical supervision: A concept analysis. *Journal of Advanced Nursing*. **31**, 722–29.

Nåden, D. & Eriksson, K. (2000). The phenomenon of confirmation: An aspect of nursing as an art. *International Journal for Human Caring*. **4**(3), 23–28.

Proctor, B. (2011). 'Training for the supervision alliance: attitude, skills and intention' in J.R. Cutcliffe, K. Hyrkäs & J. Fowler (eds) *Routledge Handbook of Clinical Supervision. Fundamental international themes*. USA/Canada: Routledge. pp. 23–34.

Sabatino, L., Stievano, A., Rocco, G., Kallio, H., Pietila, A-M. & Kangasniemi, M.K. (2014). The dignity of the nursing profession: A meta-synthesis of qualitative research. *Nursing Ethics*. **21**(6), 659–72.

Severinsson, E.I. (1995). The phenomenon of clinical supervision in psychiatric health care. *Journal of Psychiatric and Mental Health Nursing*. **2**, 301–09.

Severinsson, E.I. (2001). Confirmation, meaning and self-awareness as core concepts of the nursing supervision model. *Nursing Ethics*. **8**(1), 36–44.

Stievano, A., Rocco, G., Sabatino, L. & Alvaro, R. (2013). Dignity in professional nursing: Guaranteeing better patient care. *Journal of Radiology Nursing*. **32**(3), 120–23.

Valentine, N., Darby, C. & Bonsel, G.J. (2008). Which aspects of non-clinical quality of care are most important? Results from WHO's general population surveys of 'health system responsiveness' in 41 countries. *Social Science & Medicine*. **66**, 1939–50.

*Webster's Encyclopedic Unabridged Dictionary of the English Languag*e (1996). New York: Gramercy Books.

Chapter 9

Dignity in suffering: a theological perspective

Åsa Roxberg and António Barbosa da Silva

Introduction

The Old Testament story of Job is the foundation for this chapter addressing dignity in suffering, as this Bible story may provide some theological answers to what dignity is, and what it is not. Job's suffering may be compared to what is described as a threat to personal integrity and dignity. When Job's friends try to comfort him according to their beliefs, the collision of world views becomes evident. This conflict of beliefs occurs because the friends' self-respect and dignity of merit is tied to their over-evaluated self-image. This makes it difficult for them to correctly reflect on their own views and Job's view. It is this paradigmatic aspect of Job's suffering that is of the utmost importance today. As healthcare professionals, we need sound ethical models that function according to inbuilt moral virtues and not merely by following a set of rules. Care is built on a genuine love for human beings and for each individual's uniqueness. The healthcare professional therefore needs to gain insights into what it means to be truly human and encounter each person's uniqueness from that standpoint.

Learning objectives

This chapter will enable you to:

- Learn how recent research describes essential aspects of dignity of patients suffering existential pain
- Reflect on how dignity can be preserved in practical care and acquire the ability to identify and deal with moral evil and moral good in a caring context
- Gain a theoretical understanding of dignity-preserving care for patients struggling to preserve their autonomy, dignity and integrity.

Background

It is assumed that ancient texts, like the Book of Job in the Bible (*New King James Version* 1982), can contribute to our understanding of the phenomenon of dignity. Roxberg (2005, 2008, 2011) has found that the concept of consolation is explored in Greek and Roman philosophy as well as in the Bible. She regards Job as a paradigm of great and undeserved suffering. In the Book of Job, he experiences attempted consolation that does not succeed in consoling him. But does this non-caring consolation also constitute a threat to Job's dignity?

It can indeed be seen as a threat to his dignity if, as Lønning (1996) holds, caring without respect is a potential violation, and respect without caring is empty. Job's friends intended to offer him a caring consolation (cf. Roxberg 2005, Roxberg & Barbosa da Silva 2013) without respecting him; and Job experiences their attempt to console him as empty. In a similar way, the victims of the 2004 Indian Ocean tsunami described sympathy as a way of playing down the experience of loss and gave this advice to consolers: 'Do not mourn my tears, mourn your own tears, then we can mourn together' (Barbosa da Silva & Roxberg 2013). Like Job, a modern victim, Sävstam (2007, p. 30), challenged God: 'If you [God] give me one of the children back I will change my whole life. Everything will be different. If you give me back both of my children, you can have my whole life'. Thus, the ancient Book of Job may provide some answers to questions about dignity that have universal relevance for individuals in any time and place (Mettinger 1992). The purpose of this chapter is to demonstrate this relevance.

The intrigue and Job's perception and defence of his dignity as an ethical paradigm

Job is a respected man in the society of Uz, situated in the Middle East (Maag 1982, Clines 1989, Ebach 1996, Pope 1983, Job 1:1–4). He is healthy, well off and apparently living a good life with his big family (Job 1:13–19). However, he is suddenly beset by a series of tragedies. He loses his property as well as most members of his family. Then he gets a horrible skin disease which causes infected boils to appear all over his body. In the wake of these disasters, Job's situation changes dramatically. He is now expelled from the city and has to live on an ash heap outside it (Job 2:7–8). This was where the outcast and those with infectious diseases were forced to live (Hartley 1988, Clines 1989). Job is first visited by three of his friends (Job 2:11) and later on by a fourth friend (Job 32:2–37:24), who all try to console him in his misery. Most of the Book of Job is therefore a conversation between the suffering Job and his friends. The problem is that three of the friends' attempts to comfort Job are unsuccessful. Instead of experiencing consolation,

Job becomes irritated and impatient with the way these friends attempt to console him. Their attempts at consolation may also constitute a threat to Job's dignity (Roxberg 2005, Roxberg *et al.* 2011, Roxberg & Barbosa da Silva 2013).

The Book of Job is also a special genre, in which metaphors are frequently used to describe suffering and consolation (Illman 1996, Clines 1989). Job experiences a superficial consolation, when he says, 'How then can you comfort me with empty words, since falsehood remains in your answers' (Job 21:34) and 'Shall words of wind have an end?' (Job 16:2–3) (cf. Roxberg 2005, Roxberg *et al.* 2011, Roxberg & Barbosa da Silva 2013). In Job's experience of suffering, one aspect is not to be listened to – neither by his friends nor by God. 'If I called and He answered me, I would not believe that He was listening to my voice' (Job 9:16). Baillie & Gallagher (2012) hold that maintaining the patient's or the client's dignity is an important aspect of nursing care and this can be equally applied to healthcare. The use of visual metaphors (showing a DVD) contributed to nursing staff's reflection on their own stance towards indignity and how to recognise, respect and promote the patient's dignity.

Objective and subjective dignity

Job's suffering may be compared to what is experienced and described as a threat to personal integrity and dignity. Barbosa da Silva (2009, p. 22) explains that the term 'dignity' can refer to both an objective dignity (as a value in itself) and a subjective (experienced) dignity. The latter is an experience of self-respect and of being proud of one's own value or worth and identity. The philosopher Kant (1981) describes both human autonomy and dignity as objective, inherent values that are unchangeable, inviolable and universal and which unconditionally belong to any individual solely by virtue of being a member of the human species (*Homo sapiens*) (Barbosa da Silva 2009, p. 22; Secker 1999).

Objective dignity is inalienable and non-gradable, whereas subjective dignity is an empirical concept and therefore changeable. Because it is a subjective experience, it can change from person to person and with the same person in different situations. A person living with dementia or who is under anaesthesia may therefore not consciously experience the respect or violation of their dignity. Violation of dignity often occurs with patients in mental healthcare, who are suffering from trauma as a result of violence or sexual abuse in their childhood. This category of patient often experiences disrespect, rejection, ostracism and disengagement on the part of caregivers (Barbosa da Silva *et al.* 2016, pp. 54f). But, as human beings, they still have objective dignity, regardless of not experiencing it. Objective dignity is equal for all humans; and both objective and subjective dignity ought to be respected and not violated.

As we have seen, the health professional may violate the individual's objective dignity without the patient/client being aware of it – for example, if they are suffering from mental illness or under anaesthesia. In such a situation the patient may need an advocate or a lawyer to defend their best interests. However, a patient or client may also consciously experience their dignity being violated and be aware that violence has, in fact, occurred. We assume that the normal situation is that in which there is no violation of the patient's dignity and no experience of any violence. However, in healthcare practice it is not always easy to balance the patient's autonomy (as expressed, for example, in the patient's informed granting of consent) with paternalistic treatment by health professionals which may engender violation of dignity.

In trying to balance the biomedical principle of beneficence with that of autonomy and justified paternalism, Beauchamp and Childress (2013, p. 221) make the following statement about this complex issue:

> As a person's interests in *autonomy* increase and the benefits of that person decrease, the justification of *paternalistic action* becomes less plausible; conversely, as the *benefits* for a person increase and that person's autonomy interests decrease, the justification of paternalistic action become more plausible.

Job's dignity is violated by his friends. During his suffering he preserves his 'dignity of identity' (Nordenfelt & Edgar 2005) and in this effort he also upholds his utmost objective dignity (*Menschenwürde* as a human being). What does it mean to healthcare professionals today? We argue that it may reveal what dignity is and what it is not. Three of Job's friends' self-images and evaluation of the cause of Job's suffering apparently correspond to a traditional religious doctrine. According to this doctrine, God always protects the righteous and punishes the unrighteous or the sinner. Job's friends believe he has committed a sin and his suffering is therefore his punishment from God (cf. John 9, pp. 1f). When they try to console the suffering Job according to their belief, the collision of world views becomes evident.

This conflict can be explained as follows: on the one hand, the suffering Job is trying to preserve his dignity of identity (Nordenfelt & Edgar, 2005); on the other hand, the friends are trying to comfort him out of self-respect that originates in their own doctrine or belief. Their self-respect and 'dignity of merit' is tied to their over-evaluated self-image which makes it difficult for them to objectively or correctly reflect on their own views about themselves and others (in this case, Job). This tells us something about dignity in general – for example, the healthcare professional's dignity needs to be assessed in any encounter with another's dignity (i.e. that of the patient). If it is not properly reflected on, as in the case of Job's friends, it will result in a mechanical stance from which the healthcare professional's efforts will not relieve, but will instead increase, the other's suffering.

The ability to identify and deal with the moral evil and moral good

Implicit in Job's story is an insight into how one should deal with the moral evil and good, respectively. Waaler (2011) describes the moral evil as the shadow of the good, citing Zimbardo's (2007, p. 229) argument 'that the potential for perversion is inherent in the very processes that make human beings do all the wonderful things we do'. As a healthcare professional, it is therefore important to understand the moral evil in the light of the moral good in order to acquire the critical attitude required to distinguish the good from the evil – in other words, to discern what in the shadow of the good may be a threat to the patient's dignity. In order to acquire such cognitive ability, we can learn from Job's friends who conducted themselves rightly, but were wrong in their attempts to comfort Job.

One way to avoid threatening the patient's dignity may be to keep an honest and open mind towards oneself, daring to be self-critical and challenge the views that one's self-dignity is based on. To be honest and self-critical about one's own negative qualities and attitudes requires humility and courage as fundamental moral virtues, and this is something that Job can teach us. Courage is an ontological concept, a moral virtue, a property of an ethical act, and a creative capacity (Lindh *et al.* 2010). Here it is used as a moral virtue. According to Beauchamp and Childress (2013, p. 31), moral 'virtue is a positive trait or quality deemed to be morally good and thus is valued as a foundation of principle and good moral being'.

Let us now listen to the voice of Job (21:2–5) and the threat to his dignity (Nordenfelt & Edgar 2005, p. 20) that he experiences:

> Listen carefully to my speech, and let this be your consolation. Bear with me that I may speak, and after I have spoken, keep mocking. As for me, *is* my complaint against man? And if *it were*, why should I not be impatient? Look at me and be astonished; Put *your* hand over *your* mouth.

Job also experiences God's presence as a threat – in other words, he sees a God who is monitoring and restricting him (Lindström 1998). Job tries to preserve his dignity (self-respect) by challenging God (13: 2–3, 27):

> What you know, I also know; I *am* not inferior to you. But I would speak to the Almighty, and I desire to reason with God. You put my feet in the stocks, and watch closely all my paths. You set a limit for the soles of my feet.

As previously indicated, the Book of Job should not only be seen as narrating one person's suffering but also as a paradigm of mankind's suffering (Lindström 1992, Mettinger 1992).

Job struggles throughout the book for his own autonomy, for the right to speak out about the threat he is exposed to. This is his way of endorsing, defending and protecting his dignity. Throughout his struggle, it seems that Job is trying to find some safe space to exist in and to preserve his dignity. Job is searching for a new mythical paradigm through which he can rebuild meaning and orientate himself towards life again (Perdue 1991). It is by constructing one's life-story that existence is given form and meaning (Ricoeur 1995). Let's presume that Job did not oppose the threat the way he did. Then we would probably find Job still sitting on the heap of ashes, mourning his losses. However, he denies self-pity and instead turns into a warrior, who fights for his own dignity against false accusations.

Job's story and its possible contribution to healthcare ethics

The healthcare professional encounters many kinds of people, probably as many as there are different ways of enduring suffering (Karlsson *et al.* 2010). According to the Book of Job, what is the best way to relieve a person's suffering? Job has no direct answers to the question except that he wants to be met in his own experience of suffering, not in the other's beliefs about how he should experience or tolerate it.

Job is a lonely man in his suffering. This loneliness can be visualised as a room without windows and doors. To be locked away in such a room is to be left with only the experience of one's lonely self. There is probably a strong desire to be rescued from that loneliness. In this atmosphere the friends' empty words are experienced as a double threat to Job. On the one hand, the empty words are like an echo, spoken and returning back to the speaker without any positive effect on the addressee; on the other hand, the emptiness is a threat to Job's dignity, which increases his loneliness. By the same token, in an encounter with a patient the words spoken by a nurse may sound empty. For example, a patient may ask existential or spiritual questions, and the nurse – because of ignorance or lack of interest – may devalue them by replying: 'These questions are common among ill people, but, as soon you recover, they will lose their significance. Just take it easy, you will see!' Such words are like a ping-pong ball that pops back to the speaker without the intended positive effect. The encounter may turn into a superficial conversation that, instead of preserving dignity, actually threatens it (Roxberg *et al.* 2008; Roxberg & Barbosa da Silva 2013; Karlsson, Roxberg, Barbosa Da Silva & Berggren 2010).

How can we, as healthcare professionals, create an atmosphere that gives room for significant words about how to respect, protect and promote the person's dignity? We can at least learn the following three things from Job's attitude to suffering.

First, Job wants to be listened to. The consequence of being listened to is that the listener puts the hand over their mouth (Job 21:2–5). It is human to be concerned with oneself, but when encountering suffering there is an overall rule, to be quiet and truly present to the other (Roxberg 2005, Roxberg *et al.* 2008). Second, the loneliness of suffering is broken by a quiet atmosphere of accepting the suffering and the way it is expressed without judging it. Third, Koslander, Barbosa Da Silva and Roxberg (2009) show that the element of loneliness is existential and should therefore be met at an existential level. Why? Because existence is something we share as humans and it is also something we experience as individuals. This means that we can never fully understand another person's existential loneliness. We may ask whether it's possible to understand each other's loneliness (or suffering) but we can never answer the question.

Suffering has a private, unique aspect. It is not to be revealed or concealed – only respected. The question is how to express this respect to the other? Again, the suffering Job can help us with this. Job asks his friends to listen carefully to what he has to tell them. This may be interpreted as asking them to listen respectfully even if they don't fully understand. The wish to understand our suffering patient originates in ourselves but, according to Job, it is not the main issue. The main issue and challenge is to accept the other, thereby leaving a respectful space for the other's existence and loneliness (Barbosa da Silva & Roxberg 2013).

This view is indeed controversial. The existing literature and research argues that the main issue is to understand the other's suffering. However, viewing existence as a mystery means respectfully accepting it as it is, like a sealed parcel that is all wrapped up, making the content invisible. It means not trying to make definite what is indefinite (Dahlberg & Dahlberg 2003). To respect the mystery of suffering is to accept that the door to the suffering person is closed, but may eventually be opened, giving a glimpse of the other's suffering and existence. It is the sufferer who is the 'gatekeeper' and they have the right to invite us to their suffering and existence (Job 42:5, Roxberg 2005). This is of the utmost relevance in healthcare.

Conclusion

The conclusion concerning the phenomenon, concept and value of dignity, as learned from the Book of Job, is evidenced as follows. Firstly, the way Job deals with and tolerates his undeserved suffering has both an individual or particular aspect and a universal one. The individual aspect is private and unique to the individual. Here the suffering person can truly say 'nobody feels the pain of my heart'. In contrast, the universal aspect of Job's suffering is paradigmatic and it teaches us how to deal with suffering today, despite the historical distance between Job's time and modern time.

Secondly, Job's suffering is also paradigmatic in that the essence of suffering and the essence of dignity are mysterious and therefore not understandable. This can be likened to a room of loneliness (suffering) that has only one door. Suddenly there is a knock on the door and the suffering person has to decide whether or not they want to open the door. The person knocking at the door ought to wait respectfully on the doorstep for the door to be opened. One may even have to wait seven days and seven nights, as Job's friends did (Job 2:13). When the door is suddenly opened, the quietness changes to a sharing quietness. This sharing quietness is characterised by acceptance of the sufferer as they are, and not as they *should* be, according to the pretentious consoler's opinion (as was the case with Job's friends). The whole encounter is grounded in respect for the other's unique existence as well as their shared existence as humans. Such an encounter is, according to the Book of Job, an existential and respectful encounter, an encounter that is like resting in a dignity-preserving consolation (Roxberg 2005, Roxberg *et al.* 2008).

Thirdly, the paradigmatic aspect of Job's suffering is of the greatest importance today, as we have attempted to illustrate above. As healthcare professionals, there is a need for sound ethical models, which means living according to moral virtues and not merely by rules. This is something that Job's story can teach healthcare professionals today, demonstrating how they can preserve the uniqueness of each person and develop a virtuous heart filled with love for humanity.

The healthcare professional needs to gain insights into what it is to be truly human and encounter each person's uniqueness from that standpoint. The Book of Job should therefore be included in healthcare education, since it highlights the importance of dignity, ethics and personal vulnerability. This knowledge should be included in general guidelines and policies for all those who care for vulnerable people.

Chapter summary

- Job's story can help healthcare professionals identify, respect, protect and promote patients' struggle to preserve their human dignity

- It teaches us to be aware that a person's objective and inherent dignity can be violated without the person being aware of this. In such a case, and when it is a patient's dignity that is violated, the patient needs an advocate to defend them.

- Healthcare professionals should also be aware that a patient may experience their dignity being violated when this is not actually the case. When this happens, it is the healthcare professionals who need an advocate to defend them against patients' false accusations.

- Job's interaction with his friends can be interpreted in either of two ways: as a violation of Job's dignity, from Job's point of view; or as Job's false accusation of his friends. Violation of dignity often seems to happen in mental healthcare of patients suffering from trauma as a result of violence or sexual abuse in their childhood (Barbosa da Silva *et al.* 2016, pp. 54f).

Suggested reading

For more in-depth understanding, you are encouraged to read:

Barbosa da Silva, A. (2009). 'Autonomy, Dignity and Integrity in Health Care Ethics' in H.S. Aasen, R. Halvorsen & Barbosa da Silva, A. (eds) *Human Rights, Dignity and Autonomy in Health Care and Social Services: Nordic Perspective.* Antwerp, Oxford and Portland: Intersentia. pp. 13–52.

Aasen, H.S. (2009). 'Autonomy, Human Dignity and Treatment of Individuals with Cognitive Impairment' in H.S. Aasen, R. Halvorsen & Barbosa da Silva, A. (eds) *Human Rights, Dignity and Autonomy in Health Care and Social Services: Nordic Perspective.* Antwerp, Oxford and Portland: Intersentia. pp. 105–127.

Eriksson, K. (2006). *The Suffering Human Being.* Chicago: Nordic Chicago Press.

The Convention for the Protection of Human Rights and Dignity of the Human Being with regard to the Application of Biology and Medicine. Convention on Human Rights and Biomedicine (1997).

References

Baillie, L. & Gallagher, A. (2012). Raising awareness of patient dignity. *Nursing Standard.* **27**(5), 44–49.

Barbosa da Silva, A. & Hagen, M. B. (2016). 'Etikk og menneskesyn for en helhetlig traumebevisst omsorg' ['Ethics and view of the human being for a trauma-informed treatment' in M.B. Hagen, A. Barbosa da Silva & M. Thelle (eds) *Traumebevisst omsorg i psykisk helsearbeid – fra et tilknytningsteoretiskperspektiv [Trauma-informed treatment in mental health work – from the perspective of attachment theory].* Oslo: Universitetsforlaget. pp. 45–58.

Barbosa da Silva, A. (2009). 'Autonomy, dignity andintegrity in health care ethics' in H.S. Aasen, R. Halvorsen & Barbosa da Silva, A. (eds) *Human Rights, Dignity and Autonomy in Health Care and Social Services: Nordic Perspective.* Antwerp, Oxford and Portland: Intersentia. pp. 13–52.

Beauchamp, T.L. & Childress, J.F. (2013). *Principles of Biomedical Ethics.* Oxford: Oxford University Press.

Clines, D.J.A. (1989). Job 1–20 (Word Biblical Commentary). Dallas: Word Books Texas.

Dahlberg, H. & Dahlberg, K. (2003). To not make definite what is indefinite: A phenomenological analysis of perception and its epistemological consequences in human science research. *The Humanistic Psychologist.* **31**(4), 34–50.

Ebach J. (1996). *Streiten mit Gott: Hiob. Hiob 1–20 [Arguing with God: Job. Job 1–20].* Neukirchen-Vluyn, Neukirchener Verlag des Erziehungsvereins GmbH.

Gallagher, K.T. (1962). *The philosophy of Gabriel Marcel.* New York: Fordham University Press.

Hartley, J.E. (1988). The Book of Job (The New International Commentary on the Old Testament). Grand Rapids, Michigan: William. B. Eerdmans Publishing Company.

Illman, K.-J. (1996). *I Jobs tecken. Europa och judarna. Religionsvetenskapliga skrifter nr.31. [In Job's signs. Europe and the Jews. Scientific writings on religion No. 31].* Finland, Åbo: Åbo Akademi.

Kant, I. (1981). *Groundwork for the Metaphysics of Morals.* 2nd edn. Indianapolis and Cambridge: Hackett Publishing Company.

Karlsson, M., Roxberg Å., Barbosa da Silva, A. & Berggren, I. (2010). Community nurses' experiences of ethical dilemmas in palliative care: A Swedish study. *International Journal of Palliative Nursing.* **16**(5), 224–31.

Koslander, T., Barbosa da Silva, A. & Roxberg, Å. (2009). Existential and spiritual needs in mental health care. An ethical and holistic perspective. *Journal of Holistic Nursing.* **27**(1), 34–42.

Lindh, I-B, Barbosa da Silva, A., Berg A. & Severinsson E. (2010). Norway Courage and nursing practice: A theoretical analysis. *Nursing Ethics.* **17**(5), 551–565.

Lindström F. (1992). Gud och det onda i Jobs bok. I Aneer G., Cöster H., Lindström F. Lidande och Död. Institutionen för Religionsvetenskap ['God and evil in the book of Job' in G. Aneer, H. Coster, & F. Lindstrom (eds) *Suffering and death. Department of Religious Studies]* No. 2, Göteborg: Göteborgs universitet. pp. 25–43.

Lindström, F. (1998). *Det sårbara livet. Livsförståelse och gudserfarenhet i Gamla testamentet. [The vulnerable life. Understanding of life and the experience of God in the Old Testament]* Lund: Arcus förlag.

Lønning, I. (1996). 'Kunnskap er makt' – Etikk, verdivalg og prioriteringer i helsepolitikk' ['The power of knowledge – Ethics, value choice and priority in health politics']. In T. Bjerkreim, J. Mathisen, R. og Nord (red.) *Visjon, viten og virke [Vision, knowledge and action]*. Oslo: Universitetsforlaget. pp. 67–78.

Maag, V. (1982). *Hiob. Wandlung und Verarbeitung des Problems in Novelle, Dialogdichtung und Spätfassungen. [Job. Conversion and processing of the problem in short story, poetry and dialogue late versions]*. Göttingen: Vandenhoeck & Ruprecht.

Mettinger, T.N.D. (1992). 'The God of Job: Avenger, tyrant, or victor?' in L.G. Perdue & C.W. Gilpin (eds) *The Voice from the Whirlwind. Interpreting the Book of Job.* Nashville: Abingdon Press. pp. 39–49.

New King James Version Bible (1982). Nashville: Thomas Nelson Books.

Nordenfeldt, L. & Edgar, A. (2005). The four notions on dignity. *Quality in Ageing – Policy, Practice and Research.* **6**(1), 17–21.

Perdue, L.G. (1991). *Wisdom in Revolt. Metaphorical theology in the Book of Job.* Sheffield: The Almond Press.

Pope, M.H. (1983). *Job. Introduction, translation and notes.* (The Anchor Bible). Garden City, New York: Doubleday.

Ricoeur (1995). *Figuring the sacred. Religion, narrative and imagination.* Minneapolis: Fortress Press.

Roxberg, Å. (2005). *Vårdande och icke-vårdande tröst [Caring and non-caring consolation]* Akademisk avhandling. (PhD Thesis) Finland: Åbo Academy.

Roxberg, Å. & Barbosa da Silva, A. (2013). The 2004 Indian Ocean Tsunami Catastrophe, its survivors, Job and the universal features of suffering A theoretical study. *Journal of Religion and Health.* **52**, 4. Published online 18 January 2014. doi10.1007/s10943-013-9815-x.

Roxberg, Å., Eriksson, K., Rehnsfeldt, A. & Fridlund, B. (2008). The meaning of consolation as experienced by nurses in a home-care setting. *Journal of Clinical Nursing.* **17**(8), 1079–87.

Roxberg, Å., Brunt, D., Rask, M. & Barbosa da Silva, A. (2011). Where can I find consolation? A theoretical analysis of the meaning of consolation as experienced by Job in the Book of Job in the Hebrew Bible. *Journal of Religion and Health.* doi 10.1007/s0943-011-9459-7.

Sävstam, M. (2007). *När livet stannar. En berättelse om att överleva. [When life comes to a halt. A story about surviving].* Stockholm: Bonnier.

Secker, B. (1999). The appearance of Kant's deontology in contemporary Kantianism: Concepts of patient autonomy in bioethics. *Journal of Medicine and Philosophy.* **24**(1), 43–66.

Waaler, G. (2011). Ondskapens akse – hvor går den? [The Axis of Evil – where does its line go?] *Pacem.* **14**, 5–30.

Zimbardo, P. (2007). *The Lucifer Effect. How Good People turn Evil.* London: Rider.

Chapter 10

Learning dignity by involvement

Britt Øvrebø Haugland

Introduction

The purpose of this chapter is to show how students in nursing and other healthcare professions can learn dignity-promoting care, by involving themselves in activities that are important for the individual receiving care. The educational perspective is based on the philosophy that the learning of dignity-promoting care takes place through discoveries and experience in learning situations in practice. The subject is illustrated by a narrative about how Anne, a first-year nursing student, learned dignity-promoting care during her nursing home placement. While meeting Mrs Peterson, a nursing home resident, as a fellow human being, and getting involved in activities Mrs Peterson found meaningful, Anne changed her focus from being concerned about how to perform procedures, towards meeting the person as a whole. She discovered that they had more in common than what separated them, despite differences in age and life experience.

Aiming to develop increased understanding of this dignity-promoting interaction, the narrative is also discussed in the light of Jacobson's (2009a) taxonomy of dignity.

Learning objectives

This chapter will enable you to:

- Learn how dignity-promoting care requires involvement in each patient's focus of interest
- Reflect on how both intellectual and emotional processes are involved in the process of learning dignity-promoting care by discovery
- Gain insight into how dignity-promoting care must be person-centred and adapted to each individual.

Background

There is a need for healthcare students to learn about dignity and how to promote dignity in professional care. *The International Code of Ethics for Nurses* (ICN 2012) underlines how respect for human rights, the right to life and choice, to dignity and to be treated with respect are all inherent in nursing. Moreover, ICN (2012) encourages educators to provide learning and teaching opportunities that foster and promote ethical values in the nursing students.

In Norway the national framework for nursing education is based upon shared values with other types of healthcare education, such as physiotherapy, occupational therapy and social work, and states that (Norwegian Ministry of Education and Research 2008, p. 7):

> The basis for all nursing, respect for individual human life and dignity. Nursing should be based on compassion, care and respect for fundamental human rights. Students will after graduation have the competence to: safeguard the individual patient's integrity, including the right to receive comprehensive care, the right to participation and the right not to be violated.

On the basis of international and national goals for health education, it is crucial to teach students about dignity-promoting care as an important ethical value in healthcare, both in theory and in clinical practice. Dignity in nursing and healthcare has been defined by Fenton and Mitchell as follows (2002, p. 21):

> Dignity is a state of physical, emotional and spiritual comfort, with each individual valued for his or her uniqueness and his or her individuality celebrated. Dignity is promoted when individuals are enabled to do the best within their capabilities, exercise control, make choices and feel involved in the decision-making that underpins their care.

This definition is holistic because it takes into account the safeguarding of the whole person. Dignity-promoting care recognises human individuality and the resources of each human being. Dignity researcher Chochinov (2002) underscores how dignity can vary from patient to patient, as each one is unique. Because dignity is a multi-faceted phenomenon, its complexity cannot be captured in a single sentence. Nora Jacobson (2009a) illuminates how healthcare workers can promote or violate dignity among their patients. Examples of dignity promotion may include work that enables a person to enhance their capacities and develop their own resources and competencies. Such work may also include advocating and standing up for the person, and providing moral support in difficult situations. On the other hand, Jacobson (2009a) also quotes examples of dignity-violation, such as objectifying an individual, and threatening or intimidating or denying the individual basic life necessities. It is important to teach healthcare students the importance of ethical dilemmas (ICN 2012) so that they can become aware of situations that promote dignity and uncover situations that violate patient dignity. Many of these situations are closely linked to the work culture that exists in particular healthcare institutions and they are not always obvious or easy to identify. It is therefore crucial that healthcare professionals receive the necessary training to gain an understanding of how to treat vulnerable people with dignity, as well as being able to discover undignified conditions in a caring context.

Most of the research on patient dignity relates to interactions between patients and healthcare professionals within healthcare practice. There is very little research on how to educate students in the various healthcare professions on how to maintain and promote patient dignity. Nevertheless, the literature claims that dignity-promoting care is already embedded in the curriculum of superior nursing care. For example, White (2012) argues:

> Dignity is not 'delivered', but is an integral aspect of a nurse's role, part of which means being able to foster feelings of value and self-worth in every patient and having the ability to encompass mutual respect. Nurse educators need to ensure nursing programs not only have dignity embedded in them, but also that the humanization of healthcare is an everyday focus. I strongly believe higher education provides the knowledge and skills needed to be able to offer care that respects the dignity of patients and that an essential component of this education journey is the role modeling offered.

Dignity researcher Gallagher (2004) emphasises the importance of learning dignity promotion by reflecting on personal experiences. She suggests using case studies or vignettes in the students' education to give them 'a flavor of the significant practice implications of dignity' (Gallagher 2004, p. 594). She also states that dignity comes from respecting oneself and showing respect for others.

Jacobson (2009a) points out that dignity promotion is more likely to occur when the health professional is compassionate, patient, kind, sensitive, understanding and open-minded. In order to promote dignity, Seedhouse and Gallagher (2002) recommend that healthcare professionals try to use their own sense of dignity to act in the other person's best interest. Tranvåg, Petersen and Nåden (2013) emphasise caregiver compassion as a crucial foundation for dignity-preserving care among people with dementia.

Gustin and Wagner (2013) have researched clinical nursing teachers' understanding of self-compassion as a source for compassionate care. They identified five main elements in using one's own experience and understanding of self-compassion in order to help one care for vulnerable individuals. The five main aspects include:

- Giving one's full attention
- Showing respect for human vulnerability
- Being non-judgemental
- Giving a voice to things that need to be said and heard
- Being able to accept the gift of compassion from others.

Their findings show that compassionate care is a mutual process, which can be developed through reciprocal caregiver–patient relationships. Rudolfsson and Berggren (2012) also emphasise the value of helping nursing students develop their understanding of their patients as human beings. As a consequence, education should stimulate the compassionate self in each healthcare student. This can be done through an experimental, reflective learning process, to help increase their understanding of themselves and others. However, developing a compassionate self presupposes student willingness to involve themselves in the lives of their patients.

A survey conducted in the UK by the Royal College of Nursing (2008), including 2,047 respondents, found that the respondents remembered learning about dignity in their nursing education. They also recognised the importance of dignity. However, the greatest impact on their learning experience was observed when practical placement was combined with supervision. After initial teaching in the classroom, the students continued to develop their understanding of dignity in professional practice during their placements. Their development seems to have been influenced by experience, good role models and feedback from patients.

Goodman (2013) suggests a five-step approach for teaching dignity promotion to nursing students. These steps include using real-life case studies to illustrate and reflect upon, discuss and exchange perspectives, while applying research, policies, codes of practical review and different nursing models, as well as analysing what constitutes good practice and poor practice. As both Goodman (2013) and Gallagher (2004) suggest, real-life case studies are very helpful when learning about dignity-promoting care.

My own view is that there should be a short introductory period, allowing time for mental preparation at the university, before the students start their clinical practice. However, reading case studies can never replace students' involvement in real-life patient situations. Below is a narrative describing how one nursing student, Anne, learned how dignity could be promoted in a caring context. The text describes how she involved herself in an elderly woman's life, by 'putting herself in this nursing home resident's shoes' – making discoveries – while observing her patient, as well as her own reactions, in real-life situations. I would argue that real-life case studies are most effective when students reflect upon their own experiences. As shown in the narrative, pedagogical principles stimulate the reflections of each student.

Learning that dignity-promoting care needs to be person-centred

As Fenton and Mitchell (2002) comment, 'individuality is an important aspect of dignity.' This statement is also supported by Jacobson (2009b) as well as Chochinov (2002). In relation to dignity-promoting care, it is crucial that students learn that care cannot be generalised, but must be tailored to each individual. The concepts of dignity-promoting care and person-centred care are closely connected. According to Morgan and Yoder's concept analysis (2012, p. 3), respect, autonomy and empowerment are some of the positive outcomes attributed to person-centred care (PCC):

> PCC is a holistic (bio-psychosocial-spiritual) approach to delivering care that is respectful and individualised, allowing negotiation of care, and offering choice through a therapeutic relationship where persons are empowered to be involved in health decisions at whatever level is desired by that individual who is receiving care.

Central elements in both PCC and dignity promotion are the relational aspect, involvement and empowering the person in need of care (Jacobson 2010, Galloway 2011). In a therapeutic relationship, the receiver of healthcare needs to be involved in the care being delivered. Likewise, healthcare professionals should be willing to involve themselves in matters that are important to the recipient (Galloway 2011).

Although education in nursing as well as allied healthcare professions emphasises that the focus should be upon the resident, ethics and holistic care, students often become socialised into institutional cultures emphasising procedures and systems. It is therefore crucial that nursing education facilitates learning situations that help each student develop basic professional identities which promote values embodying dignity-promoting care, including the philosophy of PCC. Benner, Sutphen, Leonard and Day (2010) argue that nursing education needs a radical transformation – changing the focus from an emphasis on socialisation and role-taking to an emphasis on formation. Central to the formation process is personal and professional transformation through nursing education, both in theory and practice. Relational skills are best learned when students involve themselves with patients, their families and other professionals.

Learning perspective

The learning perspective in this chapter focuses on learning by discovering, and is also influenced by experiential and situated learning. According to Kvalsund (Allgood & Kvalsund 2005) and Grendstad (Grendstad & Sandven 1990), the concept of discovering means to notice, grasp, conceive or see something. Everyone really has to discover the matter for themselves. Rogers (2011) argues that subjective experience is valid for a single individual, and no other person's idea is as authoritative as one's own experience; therefore, a discovery cannot be automatically transferred from one person to another. An individual such as a teacher, cannot make this discovery for the student; at best, the teacher can facilitate students so that they can make the discovery for themselves. The most important thing a teacher and an educational institution can do is to facilitate learning situations and circumstances which make it more likely that students will discover the intended lesson for themselves. Kvalsund (2005, p. 78) asserts that discovery can be both productive and reproductive:

> Discovery presupposes an active and intersubjective process which can flow into finding something which has already been there before or create something totally new, in other words both a reproductive and productive process.

One must therefore take into account that students are individuals, and what they discover varies from person to person. The teacher or tutor has a role in supporting the student in their individual discovery process. However, the teacher also has a role in promoting the skills and attitudes that are important to the educational institution. Thus, both the individual teacher and the educational institution should focus on helping each student to discover the humanity of the individual patient, and to develop attitudes and actions that are conducive to promoting the patient's dignity. Grendstad (1990) calls this learning processes confluent (from the Latin *confluare*, meaning a flowing together of two or more streams). In this way, the individual student's discovery process (both intellectual and emotional), the educational goals of teaching and the student's dignity-promoting care are all 'flowing together'. Confluent learning is actually more than intellectual learning. It stimulates intrapersonal processes within each student, aiming to increase individual awareness of how cognitive, emotional, as well as physical/bodily reactions can forward 'learning by discovery' and a deeper understanding of the subject.

Most healthcare education takes place in clinical practice, where students receive experience of working with sick and otherwise vulnerable people. According to Benner *et al.* (2010), experiential learning and situated learning are central to nursing education. The theory of experiential learning is also central for Dewey (1987), who asserts that experiential learning does not happen in just any context, with any person or in every occasion, but requires openness and clinical reasoning. According to Dunne (1993), situated learning depends on having an environment where students receive feedback on their performance and an opportunity to articulate and reflect on their experiences.

To achieve formation – rather than just socialisation – of nursing and other health professional students (Benner, Sutphen *et al.* 2010), I will argue that it is vital for educators to facilitate effective learning situations to help individual student discovery processes (both intellectual and emotional) as an important educational goal of teaching.

Anne, a student nurse, learns about dignity-promoting care – a narrative

For almost 25 years, I have been a teacher in nursing education. In mentoring and reflection, together with young nursing students during their first nursing home practice, I have experienced their personal and professional transformation (Benner, Sutphen et al. 2010), through personal involvement in the lives of individual nursing home residents. As an example of this transformation, I would like to a present a narrative to illustrate how one of my first year nursing students learned dignity-promoting care, by involving herself in something important for her patient.

Knitting as dignity-promoting care

Anne is a 22-year old nursing student. She has been studying nursing for about half a year, focusing on human anatomy and physiology. Anne and her fellow students have also learned about the fundamentals of nursing, communication and various procedures, such as measuring blood pressure, administration of urinary catheters and so on. Before their first clinical placement, they must pass an examination and a practical skills test, to ensure their competence before meeting their first real patient. Anne is eager to begin her nursing home practice so she can practise everything she has learned.

Student Anne was given the responsibility of caring for an elderly woman who was her primary patient during her internship. She was told that the woman was totally bedridden and relied on help for all personal care. She was also told that the patient did not speak, but could answer yes or no. The first day, Anne accompanied her training nurse, learning how to care for the patient. She learned how to wash and dress her, to determine the right water temperature, how to wring out and hold the cloth, and how to turn her patient on her side in order to wash her back and buttocks. As Anne practised what she had learned, she felt that she mastered the morning procedures for hygiene and appropriate clothing reasonably well. The patient was clean and 'well cared for'.

Then Anne started to reflect upon her patient's situation: is this all? Is it enough to be clean, washed and fed? Is this a worthy life? What if I were in this situation? During one of our mentoring sessions, Anne presented this issue to me. We reflected upon her questions, and I reminded her about an issue emphasised in the preparation for her first nursing practice: the importance of seeing the patient as a person, and searching for the patient's resources in order to preserve her dignity. I challenged her to try to find out as much as possible about Mrs Peterson, including her current and past interests. She told me she had already started becoming curious about this person, trying to find out more about her. After our conversation, Anne started actively seeking to find the person behind the patient in the bed.

She read about her in the patient records. She had been married and her husband had died about six months earlier. Mrs Peterson arrived at the nursing home about a month after her husband died. She had three daughters, who all lived in another part of the country. She did not receive many visitors. She had worked as a housewife earlier in life. The patient's record did not say much about her interests.

After the next morning's hygiene care, Anne sat down by Mrs Peterson's bed, showing an interest in her and her life. She started talking to her and reading the newspaper for her. In the beginning, Mrs Peterson had her eyes closed most of the time Anne sat by the bed. After some time, she opened her eyes now and then and looked at Anne. When Anne asked her something, she nodded or gave a yes or no answer. After a few days, Mrs Peterson gradually began to respond with longer sentences. Now and then, she gave Anne a gentle smile. The patient's response warmed Anne, and she tried to use her creativity to reach out to Mrs Peterson. She actively tried to find the person behind the patient in bed. Eventually they gained more and more contact with each other. Little by little, Mrs Peterson began to talk. As Mrs Peterson began to speak, it seemed she also became more enlivened. After some days, Anne asked Mrs Peterson if she would try to get out of bed and sit in a chair for a few minutes. For the first time since arriving at the nursing home, Mrs Peterson left her bed with Anne's assistance, and sat in a chair.

From that day on Mrs Peterson began to tell Anne about her life. She used to love knitting, and was quite good at it too. She told Anne about the items she used to knit for family, friends and charity. Anne understood that knitting was a very important interest for Mrs Peterson. She also understood that knitting was an area in which this elderly individual had great mastery and long experience. Anne suggested that they could use a wheelchair and go to the activity department to obtain knitting needles and yarn.

The next day they sat down in the room, and Mrs Peterson tried to start knitting. She felt that her hands were too weak, that she was unable to knit. This made her feel very sad. She got upset when she realised that she could not master knitting any longer. Before she knew it, Anne inadvertently said: 'But I cannot knit either. Why don't you teach me?' Then Mrs Peterson explained to Anne exactly what to do. When Anne eventually learned how to knit, they both achieved a feeling of mastery, which made them very happy.

The student had learned to knit; the elderly woman experienced becoming a successful mentor. After this episode, the patient spent more and more time sitting up in her wheelchair. They took short trips outside the nursing home, and Mrs Peterson shared more about herself and her life-experience. When Anne returned to school, her eyes lit up as she related all she had learned while getting to know Mrs Peterson. Daring to get involved helped to transform Anne, and she gained a great deal from this experience. At first Anne considered Mrs Peterson just another patient to practise procedures on. Her new perspective enabled Anne to see Mrs Peterson as a fellow human being. Anne had little experience with older people before beginning her nursing studies. She never imagined seeing herself in Mrs Peterson's place. Anne stated that her new knowledge could only have come about through meeting a real person, not from a book or a classroom. By becoming involved in another person's life, Anne discovered the individuality of her patient, making it easier to understand how she could meet Mrs Peterson's needs while treating her with dignity.

Critical thinking activities

1 Have you been in a situation where you or others have treated a patient as an object? What characterised the situation? How could you have changed the situation in order to promote the dignity of your patient?

2 Learning dignity by discovering requires both intellectual and emotional processes. Mention some examples from the narrative that illustrate how Anne used both her intellect and emotions. Substantiate your answer.

3 Explain how Anne discovered dignity-promoting care by involving herself in the interests of Mrs Peterson. To what extent can a young student transfer their own sense of dignity to an elderly patient?

Discussion

This story shows how the interaction between Anne and Mrs Peterson could be either dignity-promoting or violating. At the beginning of the narrative, the healthcare professional tells Anne that Mrs Peterson is not able to speak and relies on professional assistance for all her personal care. We understand that Anne was eager to practise everything she had learned as a student. Dignity-violation could have resulted in Anne treating Mrs Peterson as an object to practise her skills on, unilaterally washing and tending to her other physical needs, without ever trying to get to know her personally. Instead, we see Anne's honest attempts to communicate with her patient, become acquainted with Mrs Peterson and her preferences, turning a potentially negative situation into a dignity-promoting one.

In her model of dignity, Jacobson (2009a) underlines how human dignity refers to a person's inviolable value in terms of being human. However, each human being also has social dignity, based on their 'dignity-of-self', referring to feelings of self-respect and self-worth. There is also 'dignity-of-relation', referring to the respect and worth shown in encounters and interactions with other human beings. In the interaction between Mrs Peterson and Anne, dignity relating to relationships is the most prominent form of dignity. This is based on a respect for human dignity and an understanding that what goes on in a patient–caregiver relationship can affect the patient's sense of self-worth and self-respect.

Without reflecting on the situation, the patient was 'utilised as an object or a thing' she could practise and improve her skills on. According to Jacobson (2009a) and Lin *et al.* (2013), objectification is a form of dignity-violation. Sadly, objectification is not unusual in nursing homes. In the everyday life of a busy nursing home, the focus is often on efficiency, procedures and systems, instead of being adapted to the individual resident or focused on person-centred care. When Anne reflected on how she would have felt, being in similar circumstances to Mrs Peterson's, she discovered that she would not have liked it at all. Anne utilised her own feelings, trying to 'put herself in the patient's shoes', then discussed the situation with me, her teacher. Eventually, Anne chose to engage herself in the life of her patient.

Skjervheim (1996) states that there are two ways of dealing with another person – either as a participant or as a spectator. As a participant, you choose to get involved in the other person's life and their concerns. As a spectator, you observe another person from the outside, ascertaining facts such as disease, function, ability, and so on, making the individual into nothing more than an object. In healthcare, it is often customary to regard patients as 'cases' and health professionals frequently choose not to involve themselves with the person. This often leads to alienation and objectification of the patient. It is not necessarily through bad intentions, but, rather, a work culture that involves a busy schedule and a long list of daily responsibilities.

Anne started to involve herself by addressing Mrs Peterson directly, even if Mrs Peterson could not respond at first. Furthermore, Anne made an effort to find out about Mrs Peterson's interests and areas she had success in. According to Skjervheim (1996), Anne chose to become involved as a participant (and no longer as a spectator) in Mrs Peterson's life.

Jacobson (2010) argues that there are two types of social dignity: 'dignity-of-self' and 'dignity-in-relation'. 'Dignity-of-self' refers to a quality of self-respect and self-worth, while 'dignity-in-relation' refers to ways in which respect and worth are conveyed through individual and collective behaviour. Anne chose to involve herself in her relationship with Mrs Peterson, giving her dignity-promoting care. This was accomplished by the way Anne addressed Mrs Peterson with an attitude of respect, showing her importance and value. Although a healthcare professional told Anne that Mrs Peterson did not speak, Anne still talked to her and asked her questions. She gave Mrs Peterson ample time to respond. Mrs Peterson started carefully at first by just nodding, and eventually began forming sentences as she felt more comfortable with Anne. According to Jacobson (2010), relational dignity has the quality of mutuality, with the potential to enhance the dignity of all actors, including Anne (a student, new to her profession).

Anne was told that Mrs Peterson was totally dependent on assistance for all forms of personal care. A person who is dependent (or is perceived as being totally dependent on others for all care) is very vulnerable, in terms of maintaining their personal dignity, sense of self-worth and self-respect. According to Jacobson (2009b), the social process of dependency, and being forced to rely upon others for basic needs, violates dignity. Nothing was reported to Anne about the patient's own resources. Anne was merely taught how to keep the patient well cared for, clean, washed and fed. However, Baillie *et al.* (2009) argue that a task-oriented culture can be a barrier to dignifying care.

Anne reflected on Mrs Peterson's situation: is it enough to be clean, washed and fed? During our coaching session, Anne started seeing the situation from Mrs Peterson's perspective. As we reflected together, I encouraged Anne to build on her own experience, and to go ahead with her discoveries, finding out more about her patient, using her own intuition and creativity, to move forward in her discovery and experience. Some students discover this by themselves, with or without minimal supervision, while others make this important discovery as a result of guidance. Some students never detect it at all. The supervisor cannot make the discovery *for* the student. At best, the supervisor can facilitate the students, so that they make the discovery themselves (Rogers 2011). The teacher or supervisor can also facilitate learning situations and give the student assignments to perform. Such assignments may include spending time with a certain resident in an effort to discover activities tailored to the patient's individual needs or desires. As students offer a resident person-centred care, involving themselves in the individual's life and interests, the probability that they will discover the humanity in each individual increases. In the latter case, students normally apply several of their senses, and feelings as well as intellect. These are also key aspects of learning by discovery in confluent educational philosophy (Grendstad & Sandven 1990).

Seedhouse and Gallagher (2002) recommend that caregivers use their own sense of dignity in a way they would assume is in the other person's best interest. Anne utilised her own sense of what a worthy life ought to be, or certainly ought *not* to be. She used her own humanity to understand another person's situation. Seeing her patient as a person helped Anne gain respect for Mrs Peterson's human dignity (Jacobson 2009a); and this conception of dignity reminded Anne that her patient was more than an object (Jacobson 2010).

Every encounter and interaction between human beings has the potential to be dignity-violating or dignity-promoting (Jacobson 2009). In some situations, it is difficult to distinguish whether an act is perceived as dignity-promoting or dignity-violating. These situations require the caregiver (in this case, a nursing student) to have the ability and willingness to empathise and involve herself in the recipient's situation. Anne started to seek and find the person 'behind the patient in the bed' by actively collecting information concerning Mrs Peterson.

According to Jacobson (2010), each type of dignity work requires the caregiver to know their patient and their capacity for autonomy. In addition to reading her patient record, which contained little about Mrs Peterson's passions, Anne spent time with her, in an attempt to learn more about her as a person. In the encounter described above, we see dignity-promoting social processes as described in Jacobson's taxonomy of dignity (Jacobson 2009a). Anne shows recognition as she acknowledges Mrs Peterson's humanity by paying attention to her. Anne spent time sitting by Mrs Peterson's bedside, accompanying her in order to meet her basic needs, and also to see her personality gradually flourish. By being present, showing real interest, conversing with and reading the newspaper for Mrs Peterson, Anne facilitated a dignity-promoting environment. According to Jacobson (2009a), a dignity-promoting atmosphere is likely to be established when the caregiver is compassionate, kind, open-minded and has good intentions. Mrs Peterson eventually responded by opening her eyes, nodding and gradually answering with longer sentences. Eventually, Anne and Mrs Peterson built a reciprocal relationship in human circumstances, founded upon friendliness and trust.

They operated not only in their roles as nurse and patient, but shared moments they had in common as living human beings. Thus, dignity-promoting care also promotes the dignity of the caregiver (Jacobson 2010). Jacobson (2007) refers to how social dignity can be divided into two types: 1) dignity-of-self; and 2) dignity-in-relation. Dignity-of-self refers to self-respect and self-worth and describes properties like confidence and integrity.

For new students like Anne, the experiences described above can help build and promote their professional identity as a future professional caregiver.

As Mrs Peterson felt safer and more confident, she revealed more and more of her personality and interests. She started talking about her life and experiences. According to the research findings of Lin *et al.* (2013), letting the patient speak about their life is an example of dignity-maintaining care. It turned out that knitting was an activity that meant a lot to Mrs Peterson, and Anne chose to involve herself in an activity her patient found interesting. According to Skjervheim (1996), Anne chose to be a participant, involving herself in the other person's concerns.

Anne became actively involved in Mrs Peterson's life, obtaining the equipment she needed to knit. However, they both discovered that Mrs Peterson was unable to perform this activity, which had previously meant a lot to her. Mrs Peterson then felt miserable, unsuccessful and undignified. The loss of her skill at knitting led to a lack of self-respect and self-worth. Feelings of dignity concerning oneself are part of social dignity (Jacobson 2009b). Fortunately, Anne immediately realised Mrs Peterson's problem, and her intuition turned a negative situation into a dignity-promoting opportunity. Through her intuition, Anne came up with an idea that empowered the patient by asking Mrs Peterson if she could instruct her in the art of knitting. In this situation, Anne utilised her creativity and showed true humility towards Mrs Peterson. In so doing, this nursing student enabled her patient to transcend her weakness to attain the position of master. This is an excellent example of social process advocacy, levelling and love (Jacobson 2009a), whereby Anne protected her patient's dignity, minimised the asymmetry between them, and honoured Mrs Peterson's self-worth.

By creating an environment of human circumstances (Jacobson 2009a), Anne helped establish a dignity-enhancing atmosphere, increasing Mrs Peterson's confidence to show more of herself and utilise more of her resources to function at a higher level than she had previously done while residing at the nursing home. The title of the above narrative, 'knitting as dignity-promoting care', raises the question: can knitting be dignity-promoting? For this patient the answer is yes, because Anne connected the patient to an activity that Mrs Peterson had previously mastered. For another patient you might choose another approach, since dignity work must be adapted to the individual and must be person-centred.

According to Jacobson (2010), dignity work may be conducted to promote the actor's own dignity, enhancing the dignity-of-self. Anne worked with Mrs Peterson to enhance her patient's empowerment. When it became apparent that Mrs Peterson was too weak to knit, Anne used her creativity to turn the situation into a dignity-promoting opportunity by asking Mrs Peterson to teach her how to knit. Anne's caring act shows that dignity-in-relation can be related to respect and worth, conveyed through attitude, behaviour and actions.

Chapter summary

- By applying both intellect and emotions (in other words, empathy), Anne discovered Mrs Peterson as a fellow human being.

- Anne changed her attitude from being a spectator to being personally involved and becoming a participant in Mrs Peterson's life. Anne developed both compassion and empathy in recognising both dignity-violating situations and dignity-promoting solutions.

- Finally, Anne discovered that dignity-promoting measures cannot be generalised for all nursing home patients, but must be individualised for each person.

Suggested reading

For more in-depth understanding, you are encouraged to read:

Allgood, E. & Kvalsund, R. (2005). *Learning and discovery for professional educators: guides, counselors, teachers: an interactive experiential approach to practice and research.* Trondheim: Tapir Academic Press.

Rudolfsson, G. & Berggren, I. (2013). Nursing students' perspectives on the patient and the impact of the nursing culture: a meta-synthesis. *Journal of Nursing Management.* **20**(6), 10.

References

Allgood, E. & Kvalsund, R. (2005). *Learning and discovery for professional educators: guides, counselors, teachers: an interactive experiential approach to practice and research.* Trondheim: Tapir Academic Press.

Baillie, L., Ford, P., Gallagher, A. & Wainwright, P. (2009). Nurses' views on dignity in care. *Nursing Older People.* **21**(8),22–29.

Benner, P., Sutphen, M., Leonard, V. & Day, L. (2010). *Educating nurses: a call for radical transformation.* San Francisco: Jossey-Bass.

Chochinov, H.M. (2002). Dignity-conserving care – a new model for palliative care: helping the patient feel valued. *JAMA: the Journal of the American Medical Association.* **287**(17), 2253–60.

Dewey, J. (1987). *Experience and Nature.* Chicago: Open Court Press. (Originally published in 1925.)

Dunne, J. (1993). *Back to the rough ground: 'phronesis' and 'techne' in modern philosophy and in Aristotle.* Notre Dame, Indiana: University of Notre Dame Press.

Fenton, E. & Mitchell, T. (2002). Growing old with dignity: a concept analysis. *Nursing Older People.* **14**(4), 19–21.

Gallagher, A. (2004). Dignity and respect for dignity – two key health professional values: implications for nursing practice. *Nursing Ethics.* **11**(6), 587–99.

Galloway, J. (2011). 'Dignity, values, attitudes and person-centered care' in A. Hindle and A. Coates (eds) *Nursing Care of Older People.* Oxford: Oxford University Press. pp. 9–22.

Goodman, B. (2013). Teaching dignity in five steps. *Nursing Standard.* **27**(27), 64.

Grendstad, N.M. & Sandven, G.J. (1990). *Å lære er å oppdage: prinsipper og praktiske arbeidsmåter i konfluent pedagogikk. [Learning is discovering: principles and practical working methods in confluent pedagogy].* Oslo: Didakta.

Gustin, L.W. & Wagner, L. (2013). The butterfly effect of caring – clinical nursing teachers' understanding of self-compassion as a source to compassionate care. *Scandinavian Journal of Caring Sciences.* **27**(1), 175–83.

International Council of Nurses (ICN) (2012). *Code of Ethics for Nurses.* Geneva: ICN. http://www.icn.ch/images/stories/documents/about/icncode_english.pdf (accessed 11 June 2016).

Jacobson, N. (2007). Dignity and health: a review. *Social Science and Medicine.* **64**(2), 292–302.

Jacobson, N. (2009a). A taxonomy of dignity: a grounded theory study. *BMC International Health and Human Rights.* **9**, 3.

Jacobson, N. (2009b). Dignity violation in health care. *Qualitative Health Research.* **19**(11), 1536–47.

Jacobson, N. & Silva, D.S. (2010). Dignity promotion and beneficence. *Bioethical Inquiry.* **7**, 8. doi: 10.1007/s11673-010-9258-y.

Kunnskapsdepartementet (2008). *Rammeplan for sykepleierutdanning.* [Ministry of Education and Research (2008). *National curriculum for nursing education*]. https://www.regjeringen.no/globalassets/upload/kd/vedlegg/uh/rammeplaner/helse/rammeplan_sykepleierutdanning_08.pdf (accessed 11 June 2016).

Kvalsund, R. (2005). 'Learning and Discovery in Guidedance' in E. Allgood & R. Kvalsund, (eds) *Learning and discovery for professional educators: guides, counselors, teachers: an interactive experiential approach to practice and research.* Trondheim: Tapir Academic Press. pp. 67–107.

Lin, Y.P., Watson, R. & Tsai, Y.F. (2013). Dignity in care in the clinical setting: a narrative review. *Nursing Ethics.* **20**(2), 168–77.

Morgan, S. & Yoder, L.H. (2012). A concept analysis of person-centered care. *Journal of Holistic Nursing: Official Journal of the American Holistic Nurses' Association.* **30**(1), 6–15.

Royal College of Nursing (RCN) (2008). *Defending Dignity – Challenges and opportunities for nursing.* London: RCN. https://www.rcn.org.uk/professional-development/publications/pub-003257 (accessed 11 June 2016)

Rogers, C.R. (2011). *On Becoming a Person.* London: Constable.

Rudolfsson, G. & Berggren, I. (2012). Nursing students' perspectives on the patient and the impact of the nursing culture: a meta-synthesis. *Journal of Nursing Management.* **20**(6), 771–81.

Seedhouse, D. & Gallagher, A. (2002). Undignifying institutions. *Journal of Medical Ethics.* **28**(6), 368–72.

Skjervheim, H. (1996). *Participant and Spectator. Selected essays: in honour of Hans Skjervheim's 70th birthday.* Bergen: University of Bergen, Department of Philosophy. nr.12, 127–41.

Tranvåg, O., Petersen, K.A. & Nåden, D. (2013). Dignity-preserving dementia care: A metasynthesis. *Nursing Ethics.* **20**(8), 861–80.

White, S. (2012). Dignity is integral to nursing, not something you learn to deliver. *Nursing Times.* **108**(11), 7.

Chapter 11

Dignity in cancer care: a discussion based on three narratives written by nurses

Marie Kvamme Mæland and Elin O. Eriksen

Introduction

Research has demonstrated that individuals who get less than optimum end-of-life care may experience the types of distress that would predispose them to an undermining or fracturing of their sense of dignity. A fractured sense of dignity may, for example, heighten depression and a sense of hopelessness. The aim of this chapter is to discuss various aspects of cancer care and treatment that preserve dignity. The chapter contains samples of so-called 'reflection notes'. These are narratives written by student nurses specialising in cancer care and attending a 60-international-credit, post-BA course at a Norwegian college. The requirement for these reflection notes was to narrate an incident from their clinical practice placement related to a patient's care and treatment.

A total of 43 reflection note narratives were analysed by both authors, who teach on the post-BA course. We found that the main theme in the students' narratives was the ethical aspect of providing care for cancer patients that preserved their dignity. As a basis for discussion, we chose three reflection note narratives to include in this chapter.

Analysis of these narratives demonstrates that the ability to provide dignity-preserving care for cancer patients is closely linked to healthcare professionals' own feelings of dignity when working with the patients. Therefore, it is important that health professionals have leaders who are motivating and who ensure the provision of dignified care and treatment. It is also important that the specialist nurse is aware of what constitutes dignity, and is able to determine whether or not the care of a patient promotes dignity. Nurses and other healthcare personnel encounter major ethical dilemmas, decisions about which may have major consequences for patients' and relatives' experiences of dignity. Therefore, it is vital to emphasise the importance of focusing and reflecting upon ethical dilemmas regarding the care of cancer patients.

Learning objectives

This chapter will enable you to:

- Use the insights of the three narrative examples to reflect upon various aspects of providing dignity-preserving cancer care
- See clearly when the dignity of seriously ill cancer patients is at stake
- Realise that the ability to provide dignity-preserving care for patients is intertwined with the healthcare professional's own experience of dignity.

Background

One of the learning objectives on the previously mentioned post-BA course in cancer care at a Norwegian college is that students are enabled to provide dignified cancer care. However, it may be easier to identify undignified care than it is to identify dignified care. Research results indicate that patients whose dignity was compromised reported a higher desire for death and a greater loss of will to live than patients whose sense of dignity was intact (Chochinov *et al.* 2002).

As teachers, we feel it is important that students develop the skill of reflecting critically upon clinical ethical challenges and the kind of care that should be delivered to a patient at the end of life. During their studies, students have the time and opportunity to reflect upon their own practice and relate it to what they have learned in class, their work requirements and their work in cooperation with fellow students. Writing reflection note narratives is a pedagogical tool and a curricular requirement that achieves the purpose of developing students' critical thinking. In their reflection notes, the students present events they have personally experienced related to the care and treatment of a cancer patient. They may answer questions like: 'What have I learned from this experience?' or 'What, ideally, should have been done in this situation to provide the best possible care?' In addition to assessing ethical dilemmas, the pedagogical intention of reflection notes is that the students explore their own experiences, assumptions and thoughts and see them in the light of their clinical practice and acquisition of theoretical knowledge and understanding (Mezirow 1990).

Dignity is mentioned in relation to euthanasia and physician-assisted suicide. In the US, this is called 'death with dignity'. In Norway, it is called the 'right to a dignified death'. This has made us wary of talking about a dignified death. Therefore, we could instead use the term 'a good death', since the concept of dignity may have different meanings for different people. Despite this ambiguity, we choose to use the word 'dignity' in relation to sustaining the 'will to live in the terminally ill', as it is called in the study by Chochinov *et al.* (1999). The way we see this issue, informed by our own experiences as nurses working with seriously ill cancer patients, is that a patient clings to life as long as possible when care promotes the preservation of dignity.

This chapter uses three reflection note narratives written by nurses specialising in cancer care to highlight dignity in cancer care and discuss various aspects of cancer care that preserve dignity. By demonstrating various aspects of dignity, we will exemplify how nurses and other healthcare professionals may handle situations in which dignity is at stake. The aim of writing the reflection note narratives was for the students to prepare themselves for demanding encounters with seriously ill cancer patients.

Why is dignity important in cancer care?

As we have shown, dignity is an ambiguous term that can mean different things. However, our position is that dignity, despite its sometimes vague meaning, is one of the most important aspects of healthcare. In the remainder of this chapter, we will link this position to some theoretical perspectives that highlight the importance of dignity.

Enhancing patients' rights and maintaining their dignity has been affirmed as a goal of the World Health Organisation (WHO) (Lin, Watson & Yun-Fang Tsai 2013). A WHO investigation in 41 countries found that most participants selected dignity as the second most important consideration, after prompt attention in care. Promoting the dignity of the patient in the hospital setting is important, and giving patients emotional support, promptly responding to their needs and maintaining their body image are vital elements of patient dignity. Lin, Watson and Yun-Fang Tsai (2013) also emphasise that the hospital's organisation, leadership and environment play major roles in a patient's experience of dignity.

The concept of dignity has both subjective and objective aspects. The preface of the United Nations Universal Declaration of Human Rights proclaims that all human beings have an inherent dignity based on the fact that they are human beings. This is objective dignity (United Nations General Assembly, 1948).

Nora Jacobson (2009) also writes about objective dignity, but she uses the term 'human dignity'. She notes that dignity has two complementary, but distinct, forms: human dignity and social dignity. Jacobson asserts that human dignity is the abstract, universal quality of value that belongs to every human being simply by virtue of being human. In contrast, social dignity is generated in the interactions between and among individuals, collectives and societies. In her research article, 'A taxonomy of dignity', Jacobson (2009) claims that every human interaction has the potential to be a dignity encounter, that is, an interaction in which dignity comes to the fore and may be either violated or promoted. For example, social dignity could be lost or gained, threatened, violated or promoted.

In this chapter, we particularly focus on social dignity, as providing care to patients affects their experiences of social dignity. According to Jacobson (2007), social dignity is grounded in human dignity, which implies a genuine respect for the human being by another human being. There are two intertwined aspects of social dignity: dignity-of-self and dignity-in-relation. Dignity-of-self is a kind of self-respect or self-confidence held by individuals. In addition, Jacobson (2007, p. 299) claims that social dignity has always been understood to be conditional, dependent upon actions and behaviour in specific contexts:

> The uses of social dignity show how this type of dignity may be insulted or violated in ways both small and large, by disrespect demonstrated in a word or a gesture; by indifference to the suffering of the sick or poor; by humiliation employed as a form of coercion.

Hack *et al.* (2004) claim that the need to optimise a patient's quality of life and help a patient die with dignity may be exemplified by the needs of dying cancer patients. The authors have systematically identified and described the various factors that either support or undermine a dying patient's sense of dignity. Their study illustrates that dignity is influenced by a broad range of interrelated variables, including pain, intimate dependency, hopelessness, depression, informal support networks, formal support networks and quality of life. Likewise, Krishna and Kwek (2014), Huijer and van Leeuwen (2000) and Saunders (1984) argue that the manner in which personhood is conceived is critical to the provision of patient-centred care and maintenance of respect for the rights, dignity and quality of life of terminally ill patients.

We find the articles by Dr Harvey Max Chochinov valuable and interesting, as, like the three reflection note narratives below, his writing deals with seriously ill cancer patients, exploring various dimensions of palliative medicine, including depression, the desire for death, the will to live and what matters to individuals at the end of life. According to Chochinov *et al.* (2002), the term 'dignity' conveys an inherent respect granted to patients preparing for death. The goal of the study by Chochinov *et al.* (2002) was to explicate the meaning of dignity for palliative cancer patients and to develop a conceptual framework that described dignity from the perspective of individuals living with advanced cancer diagnoses. The researchers found that loss of dignity is one of the most common reasons physicians cite when asked why they agreed to a patient's request for euthanasia or some form of assisted suicide.

In his review article 'Dying, dignity, and new horizons in palliative end-of-life care' Chochinov (2006), asserts that all dying patients will experience times of sadness as a normal part of coming to terms with life drawing to a close. However, approximately 25% of all cancer patients experience severe depressive symptoms, and that percentage increases with increased levels of disability, advanced illness and pain. Furthermore, Chochinov claims that ubiquitous aspects of suffering, including psychological, existential or spiritual distress, are not necessarily well understood or researched and that such distress may express itself as an overwhelming sense of hopelessness, existential or spiritual anxiety, loss of sense of dignity, seeing oneself as a burden to others, a waning of one's will to live, a growing desire for death or a wish not to carry on living any longer (Chochinov 2006). In addition, earlier research literature by Chochinov (Chochinov *et al.* 1995; Chochinov *et al.* 1998) demonstrates that patients' preference for hastened deaths increases if they are depressed or filled with hopelessness.

The authors of this chapter also find the research by Susie Kim, RN (2012) interesting because she emphasises how compassionate care is related to care that preserves the patient's dignity. In 1978, Kim was the first person in Korea to earn a doctorate in nursing science. Her interest in the concept of caring began during the mid-1960s while she was working in a ward for end-of-life-cancer patients in Seoul, Korea. As a recent nursing graduate, she became very distressed when caring for these patients. Several years later, she was deeply affected by an accidental encounter with a discharged psychiatric patient who poured out his experiences of living in the community.

In her book, *Interpersonal caring,* Kim (2012, p. 4) writes that she learned a lot about the complete stigmatisation experienced by a person living with serious mental illness (SMI), who is cut off from society and has literally lost everything, including friends, spouse, job, independence and, perhaps the greatest loss of all, their sense of self-worth and humanity (p. 5). In this context, Kim (2012) refers to 'social dignity'. She describes how those with SMIs were not treated in a way that affirmed that they mattered. This may be seen as a form of loss of dignity. Dying cancer patients and others who find themselves on the fringes of social life are more vulnerable to experiences that make them feel that they have no value and no right to be heard or taken seriously. Feeling that one does not matter any longer may cause one to lose the will to live.

In addition, Kim (2012, pp. 36–37) lists several characteristics of Interpersonal Caring (IC) that we find helpful, concrete and relevant to dignity-preserving care for seriously ill cancer patients. Among the characteristics Kim lists is person-to-person interaction between the care provider and care receiver. She affirms that the focus of IC is on helping the patient to build a sense of worth and self-esteem. A high degree of IC requires genuine love and concern for the patient, which conveys trust and hope. By discussing the characteristics of IC, Kim clarifies how dignity may be promoted or violated in social encounters with seriously ill patients.

We have cited researchers who have illuminated issues related to dignity and to situations when dignity in care may be at risk. In fact, a patient's dignity is at stake in any encounter with healthcare professionals – because those professionals may either promote or violate their dignity. This chapter therefore focuses on social dignity. Jacobson (2007, 2009) has formulated a theoretical framework that describes social dignity as consisting of two intertwined aspects: dignity-of-self and dignity-in-relation. In addition, research by Chochinov *et al.* (1999, 2002) deals with seriously ill cancer patients and identifies and describes various factors, such as pain, intimate dependency and hopelessness, which either support or undermine a dying patient's sense of dignity. Kim (2012) provides concrete examples of encounters with professionals in which the dignity of a patient is at stake.

After considering the insights contained in the following three reflection notes, we will further discuss encounters between health professionals and seriously ill cancer patients.

The three selected reflection note narratives

Each of the 43 reflection notes we studied narrates an incident from the student's clinical practice placement related to care and treatment. Students were asked to describe the ethical aspect of the incident, from their own perspective, as either dignity-preserving care or a situation in which dignity was at stake.

The authors thoroughly read the texts separately to find examples of dignified care and treatment of cancer patients, or the lack thereof. The students had nursing experience ranging from two to several years. Even though all students followed the same guidelines when writing their reflection notes, the notes were quite different in terms of presenting coherent stories.

The three selected narratives may not be typical of all the reflection notes, but they describe encounters in which dignity is at stake and in which either the patient's needs were met in a respectful, caring manner or the patient was neglected and overlooked by healthcare professionals.

Narrative 1. Nurses preparing for home care of a seriously ill cancer patient

One of our district-nursing patients was going to be discharged to his home after a hospital stay. He was to continue the intravenous treatment through a venous catheter in addition to continuous subcutaneous infusions through a syringe driver.

The nurse who called from the hospital informed us that this patient was on a new type of syringe driver, a type we were not acquainted with. As this was the first patient with a venous catheter that 'my' team of district nurses had cared for in years, and since the syringe driver this patient was on was new to all of us, we were unsure of how to deal with this situation.

We asked those who worked in the Cancer Unit if we could come to the hospital and receive instructions regarding the prescribed treatment. They were very welcoming and helpful and gave us good instruction. It was very nice to be able to come to the hospital, onto their territory. They took their time and paced themselves according to our needs, and we received good instruction. Also, we met the patient in question and had a thorough run-through with him of the kind of help he wanted when he came home.

When the patient arrived at home, he was welcomed by those of us who had been at the hospital for instruction. The fact that we home-care nurses were able to see the patient before he returned home, in addition to receiving training, made us feel confident regarding his treatment.

There was no problem in continuing with the pain treatment through the syringe driver and intravenous therapy at home. If we were uncertain about something, we called the oncology unit at the hospital and got help from them. The patient had been on the ward for several consecutive months, so they knew right away who he was when we called.

It was really very satisfying being able to work with this patient. We do not often have patients with cancer or patients who are to receive this kind of treatment at home.

The patient was happy about being treated at home in his own environment after several months in hospital. I think it was positive for the patient to meet us while still in hospital. I think that it created a sense of security in him, although he did not express it. It certainly meant that he was received by familiar faces at his home after discharge.

Analysis of Narrative 1

As expressed in Narrative 1, the home-care team's lack of qualifications may cause a lack of dignity for the healthcare professionals as well as for those for whom dignity is particularly important, namely the cancer patient and his family. For example, if a home-care nurse felt that she had not mastered technical procedures that her leader ought to have ensured that she was trained in, that home-care nurse might not want to lose face in front of the patient and might therefore pretend that she knew the procedures. Most likely, the consequences of that would be poor communication with the patient and the patient's needs going unmet. Therefore, the narrative above may be seen as a story about how a patient's dignity was safeguarded. As Jacobson (2007) noted, there are two intertwined aspects of social dignity: dignity-of-self and dignity-in-relation; and dignity-of-self is related to self-respect or self-confidence.

What was at stake in this narrative? The challenge was that the patient was to be discharged with a new type of syringe driver and that the district nurses had no experience with this syringe driver and had not cared for a patient with a venous catheter for several years. Therefore, the important issue was how to deal with the syringe driver and the venous catheter in a manner that provided the best possible care and treatment for the patient. This was a technical challenge for the nurses. If the nurses in this situation had not sought technical skill and expertise, it might have led to distrust by the patient and, thus, to unworthy treatment, which, in turn, might have resulted in an experience that lacked dignity for the patient.

One may ask: in this context, who was experiencing dignity? What if the narrative was also about the dignity of the storyteller? By being able to visit the cancer ward where the patient was being treated before being discharged from the hospital, the responsible nurses on the home-care team got instructions and were more prepared and qualified to receive the patient when he returned home. In this way, one may argue that the dignity of the nurses was safeguarded as much as was the dignity of the patient. We find this to be in line with Jacobson's (2007) research, highlighting the two intertwined aspects of the concept of social dignity. Both the patient and the nurse are individuals who need to be seen and recognised, and this story points out prerequisites for feeling confident when the caring situation moves from a special unit with well-experienced nurses to the patient's home.

Narrative 2. Lack of personalised care and treatment

Some time ago, I met a patient with advanced malignancies. This patient had been through prolonged, stressful treatments involving a lot of side effects, including severe pain, poor nutrition and anxiety. The treatment had not had the desired effect, and the patient was now entering the palliative phase. In the following weeks, the patient was institutionalised, and several conversations were held with the patient and his family. In one of the last conversations, the patient's close relatives vented their frustrations. They reported that in the time since the patient had contracted cancer they had had to deal with a total of ten different attending physicians in this hospital unit alone, in addition to a large number of nurses and other healthcare staff.

This situation had made the family members exhausted and distraught. They felt that the information they received was inconsistent and that the treatment programme had constantly taken new directions as a result of side effects, lack of therapeutic effect and variations in assessments by the various doctors.

Analysis of Narrative 2

In what way is this narrative about dignity?

The quality of life of the patient and his family deteriorated because, as an already-vulnerable family, they constantly encountered new clinicians and endured new assessments and treatments. The patient and the family were just a number for the unit; they were not treated as people with individual physical and mental needs. The family members felt that they were not worth the investment of attention that it would take for healthcare workers to become acquainted with them.

According to Kim (2012), IC is a person-to-person interaction between care provider and care receiver. In Narrative 2, the family members of the cancer patient became exhausted and distraught. This narrative is an example of the violation of social dignity. It requires a high degree of self-worth to tolerate being treated in a manner that devalues one. Since none of the healthcare professionals ensured continuity or communicated satisfactorily, the dignity of the patient and his family was not safeguarded. Frank (2014) argues that in narrative ethics, as in narrative medicine, everyone involved in a patient's care must know what story everyone else is telling about what is happening. Furthermore, he asserts that until all those directly involved in care or having claims to ethics participation can tell each other their respective stories – containing all significant details, if not every detail – only misunderstanding can result (Frank 2014).

What is at stake when personalised care is lacking? According to Kim (2012), IC means taking a holistic approach. The IC process involves the wholeness, integrity and connectedness of the person. IC is expressed through dynamic communication. In the hospital unit, the importance of continuity and dialogue with the patient and his family are neglected or underestimated, with the result that the patient's dignity is not safeguarded. By recognising the individuals involved and establishing a dialogue between healthcare personnel and the patient and his family, dignity might have been preserved.

It appears that the student who witnessed the case described in this narrative did not reflect upon the fact that she might have made a difference if she had tried to improve the care of the family by improving communication and continuity, not only by the doctors, but also by the nursing staff and other healthcare professionals. What if the department had been organised with a few nurses who had primary responsibility for the patient's care? Would the patient and his family have felt that they were being better taken care of? These nurses might have maintained continuity and dialogue with the patient and his family, and the family members might not have felt so vulnerable because of having to deal with so many different doctors.

Narrative 3 Letting the patient die

This reflection note discusses a patient at the beginning of his 60th year who was in our ward approximately two years ago. He had been in our ward several times during the last few years due to cancer in the tonsils with metastases to the lymph nodes. The cancer had also spread to the outside of the throat, where he now had a large cancer wound. This wound was located close to the carotid artery, and one side of the neck was more or less 'eaten up' by cancer. The patient had arrived on the ward a few days before because of increased pain. In addition, at home, he had had a large haemorrhage from the tumour on the neck. He had lost a lot of blood, and a blood transfusion was planned. The patient knew that he was close to death, but he wanted to fight the cancer as long as he could.

I was on the night shift that evening, and I was reading the report when the patient's wife came running in to the ward office. She said that we had to come at once because her husband had a new, large haemorrhage. I ran after her and had a thousand thoughts in my mind while I was running. What will meet me? How is the patient? Is he awake or is he unconscious? What does his wife think? As we were leaving the office, the department physician entered the ward. I gave him a short briefing about the situation while I was running, and the physician followed me.

I will never forget the sight that met us when we entered the room. There was blood everywhere. I got hold of some gloves and towels and at once began compressing the wound where the blood was pumping out. The physician made a quick assessment of the situation, and determined that there was no use in calling for the acute team. The acute team is usually called for in acute situations, but in this situation, the physician decided that it would not be of any use to call them. The artery in the patient's neck had ruptured because of the tumour. It would only be a short time until the patient died.

The patient's wife was in the room together with us throughout this time. The time from when we entered the room until her husband passed away felt everlasting, but actually it was very short (I think it took approximately 15 minutes). The patient was not conscious, and he died peacefully, with his wife holding his hand.

During the night, I was attending the patient, and his wife came back to our ward to look at him. The patient looked so peaceful. All signs of pain and worry had been 'washed' away from his face. Afterwards, during the night, I had a long conversation with the patient's wife, in which we went through all that had happened before his death thoroughly. I held her and let her cry. It was rewarding to spend that time with her in the quiet night.

Analysis of Narrative 3

What was at stake in this narrative was that the artery in the patient's neck ruptured. The patient's wife understood that it was a serious situation, with heavy bleeding, and ran for help. The nurse responded instantly because she knew both the patient and his wife and knew that just such a serious situation might arise. Fortunately, the doctor entered the ward at this time, and he knew the patient and his condition well. When the nurse and the doctor entered the room, they faced a challenging ethical dilemma in which a quick decision was necessary.

The physician decided that it would not be of any use to call for the acute team. Even if the emergency team had been called, the patient would probably still have died within a short time. The doctor might have chosen to keep the patient alive in an intensive care unit, but eventually the patient would have died, and until then, this seriously ill patient might have been at risk of being depersonalised and objectified, and his wife would most likely have had to remain outside the intensive care unit.

Based on his medical knowledge and experience, the doctor's solution to this ethical dilemma was to let the patient die peacefully, thus safeguarding the dying person's dignity. Chochinov *et al.* (2002) noted that the term 'dignity' conveys an inherent respect to be granted to patients preparing for death. The wife was present and holding her dying husband's hand, and the dignity of both was confirmed. Thus, the healthcare personnel facilitated a dignified end of life for the dying patient. In addition, his wife was able to give him a worthy farewell. According to Hack *et al.* (2004), help in dying with dignity is one of the needs of dying cancer patients.

Furthermore, one may claim that the dignity of the doctor and the nurse was safeguarded too, because they were able to be present at the sacred moment when a life came to an end. They did not have to leave the dying patient, but could remain in the room with him. Thus arose an interpersonal relationship, a person-to-person relationship between healthcare personnel and the dying patient and his spouse. This narrative therefore also demonstrates the two intertwined aspects of social dignity: dignity-of-self and dignity-of-relation (Jacobson 2007).

Afterwards, during the night, the nurse on the night shift had a long conversation with the patient's wife. She held her and let her cry. Key concepts from Kim (2012), including 'sharing', 'companioning' and 'comforting', are relevant here, in the sense that personalised caring filled with compassion occurred. In addition, the nurse experienced shared, quiet time with the widow, which was rewarding. In a sense, they met each other as human beings who had experienced a traumatic event together. The widow's experience of support and acknowledgment could very well have been important in helping her cope with the grieving process that she faced in the years ahead. Because the nurse and the widow acknowledged each other in a person-to-person relationship, one may say that the dignity of the nurse was also preserved.

Critical thinking activities

1 Having read these three narratives, specify topics in cancer care that become particularly relevant when the dignity of a patient is at stake.

2 Write a list of prerequisites that are crucial to safeguarding the dignity of seriously ill cancer patients in a hospital ward or in community nursing.

3 What can these narratives teach us about dignity in encounters with seriously ill patients?

Analysis of all three narratives

In each of these narratives, the social dignity of at least one person was at stake. Jacobson (2009) claims that social dignity is generated in the interactions between and among individuals, collectives and societies and that every human interaction has the potential to be a dignity encounter.

In Narrative 1, the dignity of both the nurse and the patient were intertwined; when the nurse's dignity was safeguarded, the dignity of the patient was also safeguarded. Ensuring that the patient experiences confidence in the competence and skills of their healthcare professionals is essential to preserving the patient's dignity. Therefore, if a nurse recognises herself as insecure when performing procedures, it is difficult to focus on the patient – or in other words, to deliver compassionate care (Kim 2012).

Currently, in Norway, many seriously ill cancer patients are treated at home, and patients are discharged from hospital much earlier than they were a few years ago. Providing the best possible care to discharged patients with serious cancer requires that healthcare workers must feel qualified to do the work they are doing. This fact must be recognised by the leader of, for instance, a home-care team. Nurses caring for patients with life-threatening illnesses face daunting communication challenges. Patients and family members may react with sadness, distress and hopelessness when hearing that only palliative treatment can be provided (Chochinov 2006). If an untrained or unqualified nurse comes to the patient's home to handle a syringe driver, the patient will almost certainly feel insecure and might lose confidence in the healthcare worker. Being insecure when performing technical tasks, such as handling a syringe driver, may also compromise the nurse's ability to communicate with the patient. In addition, the patient's family relies on having confidence in healthcare professionals.

Narrative 2 dealt with a lack of continuity and dialogue with doctors. According to the Norwegian Act on Patient Rights of 1999 (modified in 2008), the patient is the one to decide who else should be informed about diagnoses and treatment options. Still, even if a patient has allowed their family to be informed, cases exist in which physicians choose to communicate only with the patient. In such situations, family members may find it difficult to support the patient because they have been told little about the patient's illness by doctors and they are coping with their own crisis caused by the patient's serious illness and possible impending death. In line with Frank (2014), an ethical challenge or conflict may be avoided if a physician practises narrative medicine, whether or not they know it by that name. Practising narrative medicine means taking the time to listen to the patient and their next of kin, discussing both problems and options and, most importantly, listening to fears (Frank 2014; Back, Arnold & Tulsky, 2010). Narrative medicine also works in accordance with the characteristics of IC (Kim 2012).

The patient and family in Narrative 2 had had to deal with ten physicians in the same hospital unit, indicating that communication with the doctors was superficial and fragmented, something the family members resented. They felt that the information they received was inconsistent and that the treatment programme had taken new directions constantly as a result of, among other factors, variations in assessments by the various doctors. The patient had entered a palliative phase. The time when treatment shifts from curative to palliative is known to be very demanding for both the patient and their family, all of whom may experience a sense of crisis and hopelessness. According to Chochinov *et al.* (2002), patients have less desire to continue living if they are depressed or filled with hopelessness. Maintaining a relationship or therapeutic stance that is anchored in respect and understanding offers patients some protection against feeling that they have become a burden to others or that life is no longer worthwhile. 'Not feeling treated with respect or understanding' and 'feeling a burden to others' were the most highly endorsed dignity-related concerns in Chochinov's research (2006).

One may ask: how may dignity be maintained when a patient has to deal with new physicians who do not know the narrative of their illness? Who is interested in knowing the patient as a person? Would it help if one of the healthcare personnel in the hospital unit took the time to apologise and explain why so many doctors were involved in the patient's treatment? According to Frank (2014), it is important to sit down and listen carefully to experiences and feelings. If only one nurse or doctor had taken the time to provide this aspect of care, it is conceivable that the patients' family might have experienced satisfactory (if not optimal) care.

Even in 2015, this 'old problem' of patients constantly having to deal with new, unfamiliar doctors and nurses, some of whom may still be in training, is a challenge to healthcare and certainly may be experienced by both patients and relatives as a lack of dignified care. Attention must be paid to leadership – in this case, hospital leadership. For instance, lack of continuity and communication may cause doctors to experience their work with cancer patients as fragmented, and impaired care and treatment may result. Therefore, we believe that quality and continuity in treatment are prerequisites for the dignity of patients, their families and healthcare personnel (Lin, Watson & Yun-Fang Tsai 2013).

In Narrative 3, key components of IC are relevant (Kim 2012). Components like 'noticing', 'participating', 'sharing', 'active listening' and 'comforting in a compassionate way' are fundamental to the mindset of the nurse providing IC. This kind of care involves a holistic approach and the connectedness of all the people involved.

According to Hack *et al.* (2004), one of the needs of dying cancer patients is help in dying with dignity. In Narrative 3, the doctor, based on his knowledge of the patient's condition, decided not to move the patient to an acute ward, but, rather, to let the patient die. In this narrative, the dignity of both the patient and his wife was preserved. The healthcare personnel ensured that the patient's wife was able to say a worthy farewell to her husband. Chochinov *et al.* (2002) noted that the term 'dignity' conveys an inherent respect to be granted to patients who are preparing for death.

In this narrative, one may argue that the dignity of the doctor and nurse was also safeguarded, as they were able to promote compassionate care to the patient and his wife. Therefore, in line with Jacobson (2007), the two intertwined aspects of social dignity (dignity-of-self and dignity-of-relation) were demonstrated.

Conclusion

The aim of this chapter was to discuss various aspects of dignity-preserving cancer care in the light of three reflection note narratives about how dignity may be preserved or violated. The examples in these reflection note narratives all concerned patients with advanced malignancies. Nurses working with seriously ill cancer patients will find themselves in challenging clinical situations where dignity is at stake. It is important that nurses and other healthcare personnel in cancer wards focus and reflect upon ethical dilemmas and situations in which dignity is at stake in cancer care and treatment. In addition, it is important in wards where seriously ill cancer patients are treated that leaders set aside time and recognise the importance of reflecting on ethical dilemmas about providing dignified care.

If practice contributes to a greater awareness of what happens in encounters with vulnerable patients, nurses and other healthcare personnel can face demanding situations with more confidence. If they understand the importance of 'noticing', 'sharing', 'giving hope' and 'participating' in situations with patients and their families, they will be better able to give dignified care.

Research by Arthur W. Frank (2014, 2013, 2012, 1991) has inspired the way we think about storytelling and healthcare. In addition, in education, our focus has increasingly shifted to acknowledge the value of students telling stories about their encounters with patients. The three narratives presented above are important examples of understanding how a patient's dignity may be at stake. Through these examples, we have demonstrated that dignity-preserving care to patients is intertwined with healthcare professionals' own experiences of dignity.

Chapter summary

- It is important to respond to requests and listen to a patient's feelings.
- It is important to provide continuity in care and treatment.
- It is important to see the patient and their family as fellow human beings.

Suggested reading

For more in-depth understanding, you are encouraged to read:

Back, A., Arnold, R. & Tulsky, J. (2010). *Mastering communication with seriously ill patients. Balancing honesty with empathy and hope.* Cambridge: Cambridge University Press.

Chochinov, H.M. (2006). Dying, dignity, and new horizons in palliative end-of-life care. *A Cancer Journal for Clinicians.* **56**(2), 84–103.

Kim, S. (2012). *Interpersonal caring.* Seoul: Soomoonsa Publishing Co.

References

Back, A., Arnold, R. & Tulsky, J. (2010). *Mastering communication with seriously ill patients. Balancing honesty with empathy and hope.* Cambridge: Cambridge University Press.

Chochinov, H.M. (2006). Dying, dignity, and new horizons in palliative end-of-life care. *A Cancer Journal for Clinicians.* **56**(2), 84–103.

Chochinov, H.M., Hack, T., Hassard, T., Kristjanson, L.J., McClement, S. & Harlos, M. (2002). Dignity in the terminally ill: A developing empirical model. *Social Science and Medicine.* **54**, 433–43.

Chochinov, H.M., Tataryn, D., Clinch, J.J. & Dudgeon, D. (1999). Will to live in the terminally ill. *The Lancet.* **354**, 816–19.

Chochinov, H.M., Wilson, K.G., Enns, M. & Lander, S. (1998). Depression, hopelessness, and suicidal ideation in the terminally ill. *Psychosomatics.* **39**(4), 366–70.

Chochinov, H.M., Wilson, K.G., Enns, M., Mowchun, N., Lander, S., Levitt, M. & Clinch, J.J. (1995). Desire for death in the terminally ill. *The American Journal of Psychiatry.* **15**(8), 1185–91.

Frank, A.W. (1991). *At the will of the body: Reflections on illness.* Boston: Mariner.

Frank, A.W. (2012). 'Practicing dialogical narrative analysis' in J.A. Holstein & J.F. Gubrium (eds) 2012. *Varieties of narrative analysis.* London: SAGE. pp. 33–52.

Frank, A.W. (2013). *The wounded storyteller. Body, illness & ethics.* Chicago: The University of Chicago Press.

Frank, A.W. (Jan–Feb 2014). Narrative ethics as dialogical story-telling. *Hastings Cent Rep.* 16–20.

Hack, T.F., Chochinov, H.M., Hassard, T., Kristjanson, L.J., McClement, S, & Harlos, M. (2004). Defining dignity in terminally ill cancer patients: A factor-analytic approach. *Psycho-oncology.* **13**, 700–708.

Huijer, M. & van Leeuwen, E. (2000). Personal values and cancer treatment refusal. *Journal of Medical Ethics.* **26**(5), 358–62.

Jacobson, N. (2007). Dignity in health: A review. *Social Science and Medicine.* **64**, 292–302.

Jacobson, N. (2009). Dignity violation in health care. *Qualitative Health Research.* **19**(11), 1536–1547.

Kim, S. (2012). *Interpersonal caring.* Seoul: Soomoonsa Publishing Co.

Krishna, L.K. & Kwek, S.Y. (2014). The changing face of personhood at the end of life: The ring theory of personhood. *Palliative Support Care.* Epub ahead of print.

Lin, Y.P., Watson, R. & Tsai, Y.F. (2013). Dignity in care in the clinical setting: A narrative review. *Nursing Ethics.* **20**(2), 168–77.

Mezirow, J. (1990). *Fostering critical reflection in adulthood: A guide to transformative and emancipatory learning.* San Francisco: Jossey-Bass, Inc.

Saunders, C. (1984). 'The philosophy of terminal care' in C. Saunders & N. Sykes (eds) *The management of terminal malignant disease.* Baltimore: CRC Press. pp. 232–42.

United Nations General Assembly (1998) Universal Declaration of Human Rights (reprint of United Nations General Assembly Resolution, 1948). *The Journal of the American Medical Association (JAMA).* **280**(5), 469.

Chapter 12

A story of facilitators' experiences of the Excellence in Practice Accreditation Scheme and its influence on quality, dignity and respect

Robert McSherry, Karen Grimwood and Kevin Stubbings

Introduction

This chapter presents a narrative by facilitators of the Excellence in Practice Accreditation Scheme, exploring the scheme's influence on participating healthcare professionals and users/carers. The authors have reflected upon 10 years of engaging in final Excellence in Practice Accreditation, and reviewing reports and supporting documentary evidence. The chapter offers key constructs of what a compassionate healthcare organisation culture and working environment is and is not – in terms of ensuring a dignified, safe, caring and learning workplace. These constructs will be presented and reviewed against Nordenfelt and Edgar's (2005) notions of dignity.

Learning objectives

This chapter will enable you to:

- Articulate what excellence in practice is and isn't and how this model is not only desirable but achievable in clinical practice
- Reflect on why storytelling is an important aspect of excellence in practice
- Highlight why and where dignity and respect are associated with demonstrating excellence in practice.

Background

The authors have over sixty years of combined experience in facilitating clinical and non-clinical healthcare teams and organisations to innovate and change by applying the principles of practice development. Our work is 'essentially about questioning practice in the context of evidence to support what it is we as practitioners do, why we do it so and how it can be done differently' (Hynes 2004, p. 2). We would argue that excellence in practice isn't only desirable – it's achievable. In our opinion, excellence in practice isn't about working longer or even harder. Rather, it is about becoming 'smarter' in bringing innovation, creativity and flair into the organisational culture and working environment. This requires effective leaders and managers who are prepared to embrace improvement and change in the workplace (McSherry *et al.* 2003).

Excellence, quality and demonstrating quality are at the forefront of the international healthcare agenda for several reasons. Excellence is about sharing and celebrating success with healthcare workers, patients, carers and other significant stakeholders regarding how successful innovation, improvement and change have enhanced the quality of health, wellbeing, peaceful death and the services provided to local communities. At the same time, it is not only about how compassionate staff are to the patients and carers but also how compassionate an entire organisation is and how it values its staff. Excellence is about integrating the physical, psychological, spiritual, emotional and social aspects of care to create an organisational healthcare culture and working environment that recognises, respects and values the individual and their unique contribution in striving to provide holistic, therapeutic person-centred care. We argue that the vast majority of healthcare workers want to provide the best possible care and services to their patients/carers, while making their working environment and culture a happier, safer, more compassionate one.

Globally, healthcare leaders and managers face the challenge of achieving a balance between providing safe, good-quality and compassionate care while also ensuring value for money. In our experience, the cheapest is not always necessarily the best, and it does not cost anything to treat an individual with dignity and respect. These are learnt and shared individual attitudinal and behavioural aspects of each person that may have the most profound impact and outcomes.

Treating an individual with dignity and respect should be regarded as an integral part of everyone's role and responsibility. Essentially, dignity and respect should be preserved at all costs. They are not adjuncts to person-centred care but integral parts of patient safety, quality and governance systems and processes. Preservation of dignity and respect should be implicit in all organisational cultures, attitudes and behaviours, influencing each individual, shaping systems and processes. Putting the patient first and regarding each one as a very important patient (VIP) must be the central focus for all those working in health and social care.

Unfortunately, increasing numbers of independent inquiries and reports are revealing the absence of dignity and respect – in some cases even leading to neglect and abuse. Kirkup, reporting on the Morecambe Bay NHS Trust investigation (2015, p. 141), refers to 'Mounting information in terms of concerns and the general safety, privacy, dignity that patients were being afforded'. Meanwhile, the Francis report on the Mid-Staffordshire scandal (2013) comments that 'Privacy and dignity, even in death, were denied' (p. 13) and 'Large numbers of patients were left unprotected, exposed to risk, and subjected to quite unacceptable risks of harm and indignity over a period of years' (p. 25).

Regrettably, as is so often the case, it is the bad news that grabs the press headlines, rather than comments highlighting excellence in practice, such as the following:

Staff were brilliant

'The service and treatment we received in each part of the hospital was outstanding, caring and considerate thank you. Every single member of staff we met today introduced themselves and explained their role and then did what they told us they would' (Northern General Hospital 2015).

Hospital staff win award for pioneering patient service

'They won the regional Medipex NHS Innovation Awards for establishing a new, in-house manufacturing unit that creates custom-made devices for children and adults who need specialist support or stability for their bones and joints' (*The Star* 2015).

We all have to appreciate the fact that healthcare is a highly dynamic, complex and multi-dimensional system that is constantly evolving and adapting. Resources, staffing and finances are finite. Therefore, to maximise safety and quality, it is important for individuals to embrace change. Change is not always welcomed; indeed, it is often regarded as a threat rather than an opportunity and is always seen as someone else's responsibility. We would argue that we all have a responsibility, as part of our accountability and contract of employment, to seek out and use innovation, enterprise and new technologies (digital, robotics and so on) to advance medicine, nursing and allied healthcare in order to improve the safety, quality and delivery of services. This should be done in conjunction with existing policies, procedures and governance systems and processes.

In our work, we have supported individuals in building their confidence and encouraged them to see that, as part of their accountability, 'they' and/or 'people' are the ones who can make the difference in creating an effective organisational culture and working environment that is either high and low performing (McSherry *et al.* 2013, Davies & Mannion 2013, Mannion *et al.* 2005). Eliciting the experiences of people working in these organisational cultures and working environments, and from those receiving care, is important in demonstrating the wider impact of their intervention on safety, care, quality, experiences and costs. From talking to hundreds of healthcare workers, patients and carers, we have realised what an important role 'stories' play in ensuring their voices are listened and responded to.

Storytelling: a critical friend to excellence in practice

Several exponents of storytelling, including Benner (1884), McCormack and Pamphilon (1998) and Gullick and Shimadry (2008), highlight how storytelling offers a means of making sense of an experience, indicating that individuals need to demonstrate both reflectivity (awareness of thoughts and feelings) and reflexivity (challenging our underlying assumptions to gain a new perspective). This, according to McDrury and Alterio (2002), is imperative if stories are to influence clinical practice.

East *et al.* (2010) argue that central to the theory of storytelling as a therapeutic intervention is the listener, who through a cognitive process will recognise the emotional value generated by sharing a lived experience, which in turn may identify deficits within their skills base. According to Connelly and Clandinin (1990), this can lead to the development of resonance and resilience in both storyteller and listener to support a healing process (stories become the phenomena to be listened to and studied; the narrative is the researcher's enquiry which supports a greater depth of understanding).

Historically, McSherry and Proctor Childs (2001) suggest that healthcare used to embrace storytelling as a way to convey humour and reminisce and, within education, to promote reflection and learning. More recently, through various healthcare departments (DH 2008), voluntary and supporting organisations (The Patients Association Report 2011), investigations and the Parliamentary Health Service Ombudsman (2011), the value of storytelling as a measure of patient experience and satisfaction with care received through healthcare interventions has been acknowledged.

Nevertheless, a review of the works of Benner (1884), McCormack and Pamphilon (1998), McDrury and Alterio (2002), Gullick and Shimadry (2008) and East *et al.* (2010) suggests that there is no theoretical framework to guide the use of storytelling as an intervention. If we fail to recognise the process of reflection, meaning, understanding and action, stories will remain mere stories and the therapeutic value of storytelling will not be recognised. The literature focuses on the narrative within a lived experience but this potentially dilutes the content, emotions and power behind the story. The importance of learning and sharing from the lived experience through storytelling is ultimately dependent on what we have termed the tri-partnership relationship: between patient, healthcare worker and carer; and/or between student, academic and mentor. This type of relationship is important in building a genuine shared decision-making partnership between the user, carer and professional, founded on the principles of trust, honesty, openness, transparency and effective communication. We believe this is the foundation and framework of a Duty of Candour (Section 20, Health and Social Care Act 2008).

> **Critical thinking activities**
>
> 1 Write a list of possible ways in which you could capture the stories of staff and patients/carers in your place of work.
> 2 Having captured the stories, write down ways in which you could ensure that the person's voice and experiences are listened and responded to.

It is vital to capture the voices of patients/carers and fellow healthcare workers to demonstrate the effectiveness of individual healthcare workers in helping to ensure the delivery of safe, good-quality and compassionate care. We have used several approaches to capture these stories, including: one-to-one semi-structured interviews; telephone interviews; discovery interviews (used by NHS staff to get patients' feedback to understand a given situation and introduce new ideas to improve services); focus groups; walkabouts; diaries; surveys; and patients/carers and/or staff presenting their stories at quality and governance meetings. Each approach has its own benefits and challenges, ranging from the advantages of gathering rich accounts of real-life experience to practical issues (such as arranging convenient dates and times and covering costs).

Putting aside the logistical, practical and economic challenges, we have found that stories provide a fantastic opportunity to assess the effectiveness of an organisational culture and working environment in delivering excellence in practice (McSherry *et al.* 2012). The next section is a story describing how academic and clinical colleagues reflected upon existing clinical and professional practices associated with providing the evidence of assurance and compliance for the rising numbers of independent quality and professional regulators. The response by the team at the School of Health and Social Care, Teesside University, Middlesbrough, England, led to the development of the Excellence in Practice Accreditation Scheme (EPAS) (Teesside University 2015). This story explains what EPAS is and what has been achieved, from the perspective of the facilitators.

The origins of the Excellence in Practice Accreditation Scheme

The Excellence in Practice Accreditation Scheme (EPAS), launched in February 2003 by Lord Nigel Crisp, former Chief Executive of the National Health Service (NHS), has played a pivotal role in improving safety, quality and care in the NHS. Furthermore, dignity and respect have become integral to the delivery of safe, good-quality, compassionate care, and this ethos is inherent within EPAS.

We developed EPAS with the aim of:

- Providing a quality assurance framework designed to enhance and develop working practice and service provision in any aspect of healthcare. It supports the demonstration of quality in both the delivery of care and the experience of care by the service user, as well as service user outcomes.

- Providing an external independent peer review of standards and the quality of care and services being delivered within a governance- and evidence-based framework.

- Assessing and benchmarking service delivery against a nationally identified set of standards that define excellent practice. It identifies opportunities for service improvement and provides a structured approach to implementing change in an integrated way, and reveals underpinning learning needs.

The EPAS philosophy encourages and facilitates the development of best practice by ensuring effective communications, interprofessional collaborative working, integrated working practices and team building in the quest for excellence. We have also found that EPAS reduces the burden of inspection and review by offering a continuous quality framework for collecting and presenting evidence within an integrated governance system and process. In addition, EPAS promotes excellence in practice by facilitating teams and organisations to focus on changing organisational cultures and working environments through team building, devising integrated person-centred approaches to care, and in designing methods to evaluate the impact of care and services delivery at an individual and practice level.

Internationally, many healthcare organisations have been attempting to provide evidence of quality services and standards to one or several organisational accreditation schemes and/or regulators and commissioners. For example, we have the Care Quality Commission (CQC 2015), the Charter Mark (CM 2015), the European Foundation Quality Management (EFQM 2015) and Investors in People (IIP 2015), to name but a few. The relative merits and disadvantages of these frameworks have been enumerated elsewhere (McSherry & Pearce 2011). These include for example, the fact that many healthcare organisations are faced with the challenge of having to duplicate the substantial effort, time and support needed to collect, collate and present the evidence for review and authenticity to several regulators. For some individuals, teams and organisations, it may be difficult to locate substantial evidence to corroborate the achievement of a standard and/ or benchmark.

All these organisational accreditation schemes are, of course, aiming to offer a guide and/or framework to compare and contrast their practice(s) against a given set of criteria for measuring practice to a set of standard(s) and/or a level of excellence. However, following a critical review of the existing accreditation schemes identified above, a team of multi-disciplinary members identified and developed the EPAS (McSherry *et al.* 2003). The EPAS consists of six core standards and sub-standards and information about what constitutes evidence, as follows:

- Working in organisations
- Collaborative working
- User-focused care
- Continuous quality improvement
- Performance management
- Measuring efficiency and effectiveness.

More detail on these standards is offered in Table 12.1 (below).

Table 12.1
Dignity and respect aligned to the Excellence in Practice standards and existing dignity frameworks

EPAS standards	Rationale	Ten-point dignity challenge standards	Nordenfelt and Edgar's (2005) 4 notions of dignity
Working in organisations	Explores the initiatives under the policy outlined in *Improving Working Lives* (DH 2002) and concentrates on team development, communication and the sharing of information	Have a zero tolerance of all forms of abuse. Listen and support people to express their needs and wants. Respect people's right to privacy.	3 Dignity of identity
Collaborative working	Focuses on multi-professional working and development as the main issue for the achievement of quality improvement through integrated team working.	Engage with family members and carers, as care partners.	4 Dignity of *Menschenwürde*
User focused care	Emphasises the importance of the modernisation agenda by incorporating users' views into the development and evaluation of practice.	Support people with the same respect you would want for yourself or a member of your family. Treat each person as an individual by offering a personalised service. Enable people to maintain the maximum possible level of independence, choice and control.	1 Dignity of merit 4 Dignity of *Menschenwürde*

Continuous quality improvement	In all quality improvement systems that have been introduced into the NHS over the past 12 years, the inclusion of improving the quality of care has always been an issue. This theme emphasises the way individuals and teams incorporate the concept of quality improvement into everything they do. This theme aims to make quality part of everyday working practice.	Ensure that people feel able to complain without fear of retribution. Act to alleviate people's loneliness and isolation.	2 Dignity of moral stature: a dignity tied to self-respect
Performance management	To manage effectively is to improve performance and user satisfaction. This theme concentrates on how this can be achieved in practice.	Assist people to maintain confidence and positive self-esteem.	4 Dignity of *Menschenwürde*
Measuring efficiency and effectiveness	Aims to demonstrate efficiency and effectiveness in practice through the various systems and processes associated with measurement, benchmarking, audit and evaluation methodology.	Ensure that people feel able to complain without fear of retribution.	1 Dignity of merit 2 Dignity of moral stature: a dignity tied to self-respect 3 Dignity of identity 4 Dignity of *Menschenwürde*

Within the EPAS, demonstrating an acquired level of excellence in practice is achieved by undertaking a 360-degree multi-dimensional approach to collecting, collating and presenting evidence that is independently peer reviewed and testified. This is achieved by: undertaking user/carer interviews and distributing questionnaires; through completing staff interviews and questionnaires; analysing documentation; reviewing recent and ongoing audits; and through evaluating care and service interventions, taking into account feedback from service users, carers and staff members.

Facts and figures about EPAS

Since EPAS was launched in 2003, two or three teams and organisations have engaged with the scheme each year (a total of 33 to date). The majority of these teams and organisations are from the NHS in the UK, with a few from independent and education sectors. The service types include: acute (emergency medicine and trauma, critical care, frail elderly and orthopaedics, diabetes, ophthalmology); community (specialist Macmillan services); mental health, including forensics, child adolescence and mental health (CAMHS), and mental health services for older people (MHSOP); and integrated services (integrated mental health service education and a local primary school).

The type of engagement was largely full EPAS support, in which an EPAS facilitator supported the team with the baseline to final assessment. The baseline assessment is an onsite visit designed to enable the team to audit current practice(s) against the EPAS standards. This includes a report making recommendations for action and improvement. The final assessment, which usually takes place around 14–18 months after facilitation, involves input from an independent external reviewer and an Excellence in Practice Accreditation facilitator, who externally review the team's evidence against the standards. A detailed report, award and areas of commendation and improvement are then provided.

Some teams and organisations requested facilitation only, to use EPAS to support service enhancements (for example, values clarification) or improve team working. A small number of teams and organisations requested consultancy for an identified/specific piece of work – for example, the development of nursing strategies through user engagement, supporting the implementation and evaluation of an enhanced recovery programme for colorectal cancer services, performance management workshops and the introduction of Assistant Practitioner Roles and Programmes to name a few.

An award is given at the end of a team's journey, following the independent peer review with one or two reviewers. The EPAS award is between 0 and 5 stars. Most teams' ratings fall between 3 and 5 stars, indicating that the evidence is substantive to comprehensive in illustrating that the team(s) are committed and hardworking professionals who aspire to achieve very good-quality patient-focused care. This is supported by the users and carers who actively participate in their own care planning and feel valued by the team. Over the years, we as EPAS facilitators have witnessed numerous accounts, some of which have been outstanding and some of which have had areas requiring improvement with regard to promoting dignity and respect.

Looking back on ten years' experience of EPAS and how this relates to enhancing dignity and respect

Looking back over the last ten years at the feedback from both service users and staff in multiple settings identified previously, it has become apparent that excellence in practice and dignity go hand in hand. The term 'dignity' is derived from the Latin *dignus*, meaning 'worthy' (Mairis 1994), and the *Oxford English Dictionary* (2002) defines dignity as 'the state or quality of being worthy of honour or respect'.

Despite the conciseness of this definition, dignity is a complex concept. Mairis (1994, p. 952) said: 'Dignity exists when an individual is capable of exerting control over his or her behaviour, surroundings and the way in which he or she is treated by others. He or she should be capable of understanding information and making decisions.' Likewise, the Royal College of Nursing (2008) defines dignity as a measure of how people feel, think and behave in relation to the worth or value of themselves and others. To treat someone with dignity is to treat them as being of worth, in a way that is respectful of them as valued individuals.

Having engaged with patients, carers and healthcare workers in a variety of clinical settings, we have found that some common themes have emerged pertaining to how dignity may be promoted and/or diminished. These are summarised, with examples from our experiences in practice, in Table 12.2 (below).

Table 12.2
Examples of the promotion and maintenance of dignity and respect in practice

Theme	Rationale	Outstanding exemplar	Improvement exemplar
Physical environment	The physical structure and layout of a ward, department and/or residential/nursing care home can have a profound impact on the physical, psychological, spiritual, emotional and social well-being of the individual, along with the safety and quality of the care provided.	Service users and carers were involved in the redesign of a new adult forensic community service.	A challenging behaviour unit for mental health services for older people did not have a garden and/or area for recreational activities for patients, carers and staff to access.
Organisational culture	The organisational culture and working environment has the potential to influence patient safety, the quality of care, dignity and respect and care and compassion.	A specialist Macmillan Team had a sound vision, values and philosophy that permeated throughout the entire team. This resulted in effective team working through visible transformational leadership.	Enhancements in a hospital diabetes service associated with engaging users in the evaluation of their care and wider service.
Attitudes and behaviour	The attitudes and behaviour of individuals and the whole team can have a significant impact on ensuring dignity and respect for the individual – for patients, carers and healthcare workers.	A mental health service for older people had a shared decision-making approach which fostered a culture based on trust where users could freely express concerns and issues whilst ensuring their anonymity, dignity and respect were always prioritised.	An independent psychiatric forensic unit had a high vacancy and sickness and absence record. They were recommended to develop a workforce strategy that would reflect future needs, succession planning and the retention of existing staff.

| Activities and performance | Activities, performance and the way in which these are carried out can impact on patient safety, care quality and dignity. | An Emergency and Trauma Department had a wide range of clearly identified initiatives that improved the quality of care provided to patients. The work being carried out with vulnerable groups (such as those suffering domestic violence and the elderly, in particular patients with dementia) showed strong leadership and a team approach which had produced original and practical innovations for the benefit of patients that had been disseminated throughout the department. | An integrated children's mental health, education and social care service was encouraged to establish the impact of multi-disciplinary staff and stakeholder input on the quality of care and services. |

The exemplars detailed in Table 12.2 confirm that promoting and maintaining dignity and respect for patients, carers and healthcare workers is highly challenging and complex. This is because dignity and respect are linked to several significant areas associated with ensuring excellence in practice, including the physical environment and the prevailing organisational culture and working environment. The attitudes and behaviours espoused by healthcare workers throughout the various activities in the area all have the potential to affect performance (individual, team and organisational) either positively or negatively. In our opinion, fostering a person-centred organisational culture and working environment that adopts person-centred approaches is the best way to ensure that dignity and respect remain integral to all aspects of practice development (McSherry & Warr 2008, 2010; McCance *et al.* 2013).

Dignity and respect are multi-faceted and interwoven throughout our complex healthcare structures, systems and processes, and their maintenance depends on human attitudes, values, beliefs, behaviours and interactions in the workplace. Interestingly, in settings where good-quality care and compassion exist, dignity and respect often go unnoticed and unrewarded. But when good-quality care and compassion are absent, the lack of dignity and respect is often publicly highlighted, frowned upon and demonised in the workplace.

From our experience of facilitating teams in their journey towards excellence, dignity and respect are usually implicit (rather than explicit) in their visions, values, beliefs, philosophy and professional and clinical practice. What we have noticed from some of the exemplars in Table 12.1, and what is fundamentally important in the debate, is that in areas where dignity is present, people feel in control, valued, confident, comfortable and able to make decisions for themselves. When dignity is absent, people feel devalued, and lacking in control and comfort. They may lack confidence and be unable to make decisions for themselves. They may feel humiliated, embarrassed or ashamed.

It should always be remembered that dignity and respect apply equally to those who have capacity and to those who lack it, for whatever reason. Everyone has equal worth as a human being and must be treated as if they are able to feel, think and behave in relation to their own worth or value. The healthcare and/or nursing teams should therefore treat all people (in all settings, whatever their health status) with dignity, and dignified care should continue after death (RCN 2008).

Discussion

In our opinion, both human and social dignity are important. The question that needs to be asked is how, as healthcare workers and human beings, we can promote and maintain dignity regardless of the situation. The exemplars in Table 12.2 offer some insight into how this can be achieved in everyday healthcare practice. However, we also have to be mindful of the fact that dignity and respect are sometimes violated and that this is not acceptable in the caring profession. Everyone needs to be treated with respect and dignity, no matter what their culture, religion, sexuality, disability or illness.

We suggest that a good way of ensuring that dignity and respect are at the forefront of care and compassion is the following. Ensure that the '10-Point Dignity Challenge Standards' (The National Dignity Council 2016), identified in Table 12.1, are integrated within every healthcare worker's professional accountability, contract of employment and job description. We must also educate and train healthcare workers to remind them of what constitutes the qualities of dignity. A useful framework to support this type of approach is available from the Nursing and Midwifery Council (NMC 2009). The NMC issued this guidance to support nurses, the elderly and their families in gaining the appropriate care. The guidance can be used by employers to measure performance and is underpinned by the *NMC Code of Conduct* to help nurses provide safe, effective care, in a way that ensures an older person's dignity and demonstrates respect. The Nursing and Midwifery Council (2009) guidance for nurses is supported by key organisations, including the Department of Health, Help the Aged, the Patients Association, For Dementia, and Action on Elder Abuse. The NMC guidance reflects the views of older people and carers across the UK – that the needs of the elderly are not always being met when it comes to the care they receive. We would also argue that it is not only older people but all individuals whose rights, responsibilities and humanity must be valued and respected, along with their dignity, at all times.

The essential skills required to promote and maintain dignity and respect are:

- Understanding of the person, their circumstances, their condition and their unique situation and individuality
- Having the appropriate knowledge base
- Communicating effectively, both verbally and non-verbally
- Being able to care in a compassionate way
- Working in a team effectively and efficiently
- Adopting a philosophy of person-centred care.

When we unpick dignity and respect within the context of the Excellence in Practice Accreditation Scheme, we can see from Table 12.1 how these concepts align themselves to the six core standards, alongside Nordenfelt and Edgar's (2005) four notions of dignity.

'Dignity and respect as merit' is about ensuring that the individual's uniqueness is preserved and respected as part of ensuring their safety, the delivery of compassionate, good-quality care and services, and ensuring a peaceful death. We would go a step further and argue that it is about adopting a person-centred approach through engaging and involving the patient or service user in shared decision-making at all times. Whether or not they appear to have the capacity to make decisions about their own care, their consent must be sought for all treatments, interventions and/or in ensuring a peaceful death where applicable. When a patient is unconscious and/or totally unable to communicate their wishes, the healthcare professional must then seek consent from their family members and carers and/or legal guardian.

'Dignity and respect as moral stature: a dignity tied to self-respect' is about affording the individual dignity and respect at all times, recognising and respecting their unique situation and status. We would also suggest that dignity as moral stature is about looking at ourselves, ensuring that our own beliefs, values, assumptions behaviour and actions complement patient safety, and good-quality, compassionate care. It is about challenging situations and events where dignity and respect as moral stature have been compromised or neglected.

'Dignity and respect of identity' means acknowledging the fact that, as part of the working of the organisation's mission, values, beliefs, attributes and characteristics, the individual's integrity and unique identity as a human being are always put first.

'The dignity and respect of *Menschenwürde*' is about respecting the person as a human being. From our experience, it is about focusing on the uniqueness of the individual and their situation. Care, interventions and treatments should always focus on preserving the uniqueness of the individual. Self-determination and having the ability to cooperate, as well as finding the right time to use persuasion, have both been found to be crucial dignity-preserving principles (Jakobsen & Sørlie, 2010). We would endorse Jacobson's (2009) work identifying some of the qualities of dignity and respect, and the association with the person's feelings and emotions where honesty, good intentions/acts, and the promotion of self-worth are promoted and maintained throughout their episode of care.

EPAS makes a significant contribution by helping to ensure that the individual's respect and dignity is promoted and maintained at all times. EPAS does this by implicitly encouraging individuals, teams and/or organisations to adhere to the six core standards. The following case study illustrates this in action.

Case study: a facilitator's account of the development of a purpose-built unit to accommodate the unique patient's needs

As a facilitator of EPAS, I would like to share my story of how I had the privilege of working with a team of healthcare professionals who initiated the care of the frail and elderly with a fractured neck of femur in a specialised unit.

Historically, all elderly patients were admitted to the accident and emergency unit (A&E) at the regional hospital in question. Due to waiting times and volume of patients, this often meant that frail elderly patient with a fractured neck of femur could be left waiting on a trolley for four hours plus. The staff also identified that these patients were kept waiting on a trolley, uncomfortable and in pain. If the bays were full on the patient's arrival at A&E, they would be left on a trolley in a corridor until there was a cubicle space for them to be assessed and the necessary interventions could be carried out. The dignity of the patient (in a gown, elderly and disorientated) was being compromised.

In 2009, the Nursing and Midwifery Council (NMC) issued guidance to support nurses, the elderly and their families in gaining the appropriate care. The guidance can be used by employers to measure performance and is underpinned by the *NMC Code of Conduct* to help nurses provide safe, effective care, in a way that ensures an older person's dignity and demonstrates respect.

The questions asked in this case scenario were:
• What about the patient's dignity?
• Did the staff, as healthcare professionals, show respect for their patients?

After auditing the figures recording the number of patients attending A&E with fractured neck of femur, I listened to carers' complaints about the lack of dignity afforded their relatives, as they lay on a trolley for hours, often disorientated, waiting to be treated. Where was the respect for this elderly person? Would you want your relative to be treated in this way?

As the Royal College of Nursing (RCN 2008) highlight, dignity is defined by how people feel, think and behave in relation to the worth or value of themselves and others. To treat someone with dignity is to treat them as being of worth, in a way that is respectful of them as valued individuals. In care situations (as already detailed in Table 12.1), dignity may be promoted or diminished by the physical environment, the organisational culture, the attitudes and behaviour of the nursing team and others, and the way in which care activities are carried out.

In this exemplar, a forward-thinking Trust discussed the problem and assessed what they could do to correct it. An initiative was discussed and planned and then the logistics (including the cost and an appropriate building to admit the frail elderly fractured neck of femur patients to) were established. The ambulance drivers would take the fractured neck of femur patients directly to this purpose-built unit. This meant that the patient could be transferred from the ambulance straight to the unit without having to go via A&E. The patient would then be seen straight away, and pain relief and treatment would be given as prescribed – without the prolonged wait in A&E to be seen. This unit was evaluated very well, both by service users and their carers.

This is when I was invited as an external facilitator to view the unit and to accredit the new unit through the EPAS framework for its excellence of quality and the dignity and respect that had been re-established for their patients.

Staff spoke to me about how they could promote the patients' dignity by allowing them to be cared for directly by appropriately trained staff, and how they respected their patients' wishes by giving them pain relief as soon as they were admitted to the unit. It was evident that the development of the unit had been positively received by patients, carers and staff: firstly, through the change in the physical environment; secondly, through the culture change in the way health professionals now cared for the frail elderly patients in a more direct way; and thirdly, through the change in staff attitudes and the way they communicated with A&E and the paramedics. The staff discussed with me how their care had changed for the benefit of the patient, and how they felt they were promoting the patient's respect and dignity by listening to their needs and keeping them pain free. Fourthly, there was the fact that care activities were carried out in a patient-centred way, meeting their patients' needs immediately and not after many hours of them waiting in A&E.

The patients and their carers were interviewed and they commented on how happy they were, and that they had the reassurance of being admitted directly to a purpose-built unit instead of a long wait in A&E.

Conclusion

As human beings, we should all ensure that we preserve and protect the uniqueness of the individual through their life and their death, affording them both dignity and respect. Dignity and respect should not be regarded as additions to healthcare and caring but an integral part of holistic care and the therapeutic relationship between patient, carer, significant loved ones and healthcare worker. Dignity and respect can be influenced both positively and negatively by the physical environment, organisational culture, attitudes and behaviour of individuals, and the activities and performance of individuals in their practice.

From our experience of facilitating teams, excellence in practice is not only desirable – it's achievable. Excellence in practice is about integrating dignity and respect throughout all aspects of care and services. This must include focusing on the working of organisations, collaborative working, user-focused care, continuous quality improvement, performance management and measuring efficiency and effectiveness. For some teams and organisations, the challenge lies in making explicit the way dignity and respect are promoted and maintained in their services. We have found that dignity and respect are often implied but not often made explicit, and are sometimes only highlighted when enhancements are required in response to external independent review and scrutiny.

Finally, as facilitators of excellence in practice, we strongly advocate storytelling as a way of learning and sharing in practice. Storytelling is a fantastic way of capturing the experiences of the individual (whether they are a patient, carer or healthcare worker) and of a team. This 'captured narrative' (and/or account of a real, personal experience) can then be used to highlight how person-centred we are in our approach to caring.

Chapter summary

- Excellence in practice isn't only desirable – it's achievable.
- It does not cost anything to treat an individual with dignity and respect.
- From our experience, dignity and respect apply equally to those who have capacity and to those who lack it.
- Storytelling is a means of making sense of an experience indicating that individuals need to demonstrate both reflectivity (awareness of thoughts and feelings) and reflexivity (challenging our underlying assumptions to gain a new perspective).
- Dignity and respect can be influenced both positively and negatively by the physical environment, organisational culture, attitudes and behaviour of individuals, and the activities and performance of individuals in their practice.

Suggested reading

For more in-depth understanding, you are encouraged to read:

McSherry, R. & Warr, J. (2010). *Implementing Excellence in your Health Care Organization: Managing, Leading and Collaborating.* Maidenhead: Open University Press.

Moullin, M. (2002). *Delivering Excellence in Health and Social Care: Quality, Excellence and Performance Management.* Buckingham: Open University Press.

References

Benner P. (1984). *From Novice to Expert.* New York: Addison Wesley.

Care Quality Commission (2015). *The independent regulator of health and social care in England,* London. http://www.cqc.org.uk/ (accessed 14 June 2016).

Charter Mark (2015). *The Scottish Government: Charter Mark Scotland.* http://www.gov.scot/Topics/Government/PublicServiceReform/18778/15020 (accessed 14 June 2016).

Connelly, F. M., & Clandinin, D. J. (1990). Stories of experience and narrative enquiry. *Educational Researcher.* **19**, 2–14.

Davies, T.O.H. & Mannion, R. (2013). Will prescriptions for cultural change improve the NHS? *British Medical Journal.* **346**, f1305 1–4.

Department of Health (DH) (2008). *High Quality Care for All: NHS next Stage Review Final Report.* London: HMSO.

Department of Health (DH) (2002) *Improving Working Lives Assessment and Accreditation for Strategic Health Authorities and Workforce Development Confederations* Department of Health, London.

East, L., Jackson, J., Obrien, L. & Peters, P. (2010). Storytelling: an approach that helps develop resilience. *Nurse Researcher.* **17**(3), 17–25.

European Foundation Quality Management (2015). http://www.efqm.org (accessed 14 June 2016).

Gullick J. & Shimadry B. (2008). Using Patient Stories to Improve Quality of Care. *Nursing Times.* **104**(10), 33–34.

Hynes, G. (2004). *Exploring Philosophical Underpinnings for Practice Development Education in Ireland.* Paper presented at the 5th Annual International Research Conference. School of Nursing and Midwifery Studies. Dublin: University of Dublin, Trinity College.

Investors in People (2015). *The standard for people management.* https://www.investorsinpeople.com/ (accessed 14 June 2016).

Jacobson, N. (2009). A taxonomy of dignity: a grounded theory study. *BMC International Health and Human Rights.* **9**(3), 1–9.

Jakobsen, R. & Sørlie, V. (2010). Dignity of older people in a nursing home: narratives of care providers. *Nursing Ethics.* **17**, 289–300.

Kirkup, B. (2015). *The Report of the Morecambe Bay Investigation: An independent investigation into the management, delivery and outcomes of care provided by the maternity and neonatal services at the University Hospitals of Morecambe Bay NHS Foundation Trust from January 2004 to June 2013, March 2015.* https://www.gov.uk/government/uploads/system/uploads/attachment_data/file/408480/47487_MBI_Accessible_v0.1.pdf (accessed 14 June 2016).

Mairis, E.D. (1994). Concept clarification in professional practice: dignity. *Journal of Advanced Nursing.* **5**(3), 947–953.

Mannion, R., Davies, H.T.O. & Marshall, N.M. (2005). Cultural characteristics of 'high' and 'low' performing hospitals. *Journal of Health Organization and Management.* **19**(6), 431–39.

McCance, T., Gribben, B., McCormack, B.E.A. & Laird, A.L. (2013). Promoting person-centred practice within acute care: the impact of culture and context on a facilitated practice development programme. *International Practice Development Journal.* 3, 1, 1–17 http://www.fons.org/Resources/Documents/Journal/Vol3No1/IDPJ_0301_02.pdf (accessed 14 June 2016).

McCormack, C. & Pamphilon, B. (1998). 'The Balancing Act' cited in J. McDrury & M. Alterio (2003). *Learning Through Storytelling in Higher Education: Using Reflection and Experience to improve Learning.* London: Kogan Page.

McDrury, J. & Alterio, M. (2003). *Learning Through Storytelling in Higher Education: Using Reflection and Experience to improve Learning.* London: Kogan Page.

McSherry, R., McSherry, W. & Pearce, P. (2013). Can clinical governance act as a cultural barometer? *Nursing Times.* **109**(19), 12–15

McSherry, R., Pearce, P., Grimwood, K. & McSherry, W. (2012). The pivotal role of nurse managers, leaders and educators in enabling excellence in nursing care. *Journal of Nursing Management.* **20** (1), 7–19.

McSherry, R. & Pearce, P. (2011). *Clinical Governance: a Guide to Implementation for Healthcare Professionals.* 3rd edn. Oxford: Blackwell Science.

McSherry, R. & Warr, J. (2008). *An Introduction to Excellence in Practice Development in Health and Social Care.* Maidenhead: Open University Press.

McSherry, R. & Warr, J. (2010.) *Implementing Excellence in your Health Care Organization: Managing, Leading and Collaborating.* Maidenhead: Open University Press.

McSherry R., Kell J. & Mudd D. (2003). Best practice using excellence in practice accreditation scheme. *British Journal of Nursing.* **12**(10), 623–29.

McSherry, R. & Proctor-Childs, T. (2001). Promoting evidence-based practice through an integrated model of care: patient case studies as a teaching method. *Nurse Education in Practice.* 1, 19–26.

Nordenfelt, L. & Edgar, A. (2005). The four notions of dignity. *Quality in Ageing.* **6**(1), 17–21.

Northern General Hospital (2015). *Compliments Board NGH, England.* http://www.northamptongeneral.nhs.uk/ForPatientsVisitors/Praise-from-Patients.aspx (accessed 14 June 2016).

Nursing and Midwifery Council (NMC) (2009). *The NMC Code of Professional Conduct: Standards for Conduct, Performance and Ethics.* London: NMC.

Oxford English Dictionary (2002). 10th edn. Revised. Oxford: Oxford University Press.

Parliamentary and Health Service Ombudsman (2015). *Report of the Health Service Ombudsmen on ten investigations into NHS care of older people – Case studies.* http://www.ombudsman.org.uk/care-and-compassion/case-studies (accessed 14 June 2016).

Royal College of Nursing (RCN) (2008). *Defending Dignity – Challenge and Opportunities for Nursing.* London: RCN.

'Section 20: Duty of candour' in *The Health and Social Care Act 2008 (Regulated Activities) Regulations 2014* [webpage on the Internet]. 2014, London. http://www.legislation.gov.uk/ukdsi/2014/9780111117613 (accessed 14 June 2016).

The Patients Association (2011). *We've been listening, have you been learning?* Online report. http://www.patients-association.org.uk/wp-content/uploads/2014/08/Patient-Stories-2011.pdf (accessed 14 June 2016).

The Mid Staffordshire NHS Foundation Trust Public Inquiry (2013). *Report of the Mid Staffordshire NHS Foundation Trust Public Inquiry: Executive Summary.* http://webarchive.nationalarchives.gov.uk/20150407084003/http://www.midstaffspublicinquiry.com/ (accessed 13 June 2016).

The National Dignity Council (2016) *The 10 Dignity DO's* http://www.dignityincare.org.uk/About/The_10_Point_Dignity_Challenge/(accessed 21 June 2016)

The Star (2015) Doncaster hospital staff win award for pioneering patient service. *The Star,* Doncaster. http://www.thestar.co.uk/news/health/local-health/doncaster-hospital-staff-win-award-for-pioneering-patient-service-1-7512850 (accessed 14 June 2016).

Teesside University (2015). *The Excellence in Practice Accreditation Scheme – (EPAS).* Middlesbrough. http://www.tees.ac.uk/schools/soh/epas_index.cfm (accessed 14 June 2016).

Afterword: what gets in the way of dignity, and why you must not let it

After all these stories and conceptual classifications, two final learning objectives remain. One, unfortunately negative, is to underscore what has often been missing or left in the background in the preceding chapters: all that obstructs, that gets in the way of nurses as they work to sustain patients' dignity. The second and positive objective is to offer some final testimony to how important dignity is to patients – often as important as whatever medical treatment can offer.

In Chapter 2, Oddgeir Synnes and I quote a nurse who is discharging an elderly patient sooner than she thinks advisable, with less time than she wants to teach her patient's elderly spouse how to care for him at home. 'And the pressure is on,' that nurse says (p. xx) – and it is. She knows that another patient is already in surgery and will soon need to fill the bed of the patient she is discharging. The hospital's bed-rotation schedule compels that nurse to decide how far to compromise the dignity of the patient she is discharging in order not to cause the patient arriving on the unit to lose dignity by being warehoused on a gurney in the corridor. In the university teaching hospital closest to where I live, patients can spend several days in the corridor before a room is available for them – with all the loss of dignity that spatial placement causes them (though at least receiving minimal treatment). For the nurse under pressure, the question is not whether to preserve the patient's dignity. The question is whose dignity to sacrifice in what way, in order to sustain some measure of another patient's dignity.

In Chapter 7 we hear this same issue in a story told from the patient's viewpoint. Elaine Maxwell, writing about her father's end-of-life care, describes nurses 'coming to tell me how busy and stressed they were, and how much pressure they were under to free up beds so that the hospital did not breach the four-hour waiting target for emergency department admissions' (p. xxx). The final part of this quotation matters. The government, or some higher regulatory body, has set a standard of care – a waiting-time target – that the hospital administration is required to meet, or the institution will be adversely affected. The hospital administration then sets standards for units, and the nurses have to enforce those standards – their jobs require them to do that. The nurses are thus doubly removed from the decision-making that sets the pace of their work.

The nurses caring for Elaine Maxwell's father might laugh, sadly, at Chapter 10's story of Anne, the student nurse, who has time to sit on the bed of her patient, Mrs Peterson, and learn about her life (pp. xxx ff.). Anne's encouragement of Mrs Peterson to teach her to knit is an inspired clinical intervention. Full dignity requires believing that one's life has a value that is made tangible by seeing its beneficial effects on others. As Mrs

Peterson teaches Anne to knit, she knows she herself can still be of service, rather than being only the one who is served. But how long will this luxury of time last, after Anne's training period ends? When will the pressure be on her, and when will time spent with one patient be time taken away from another?

Nurses, like any healthcare providers, have to distinguish and balance two recognitions, each of which involves honest and therefore difficult self-reflection. One is to recognise how significant their own personal, moral/ethical commitment to their patients' dignity actually is, when those commitments are confronted with institutional practices that come to the nurse as 'orders' to act in ways that risk or certainly incur a patient's loss of dignity. That issue might be called the sphere of effective personal control. I emphasise that it requires particular honesty to reflect on whether our acts reflect what we believe are our commitments.

The complementary recognition is whether or not the nurse's employer is providing the resources that are crucial to preserving both the patient's dignity and the nurse's dignity. These resources begin with time and space: time to acknowledge the distinctive humanity of each patient; and space, especially for privacy. The nurse on the unit floor has little control over these resources. Again, it requires reflective honesty not to rationalise the practices of one's employer as benign, because anyone's self-image is tied to their image of institutional entities of which they are part. Healthcare workers easily lapse into the tautology that what is provided for patients must be all that patients need, and therefore patients' and families' demands for more resources are unreasonable. Most patients fear, with good reason, being labelled by nurses as 'demanding' and then being given lesser care; that happens.

I believe that a satisfying career in healthcare depends upon balancing these two recognitions. On the one hand, personal commitments can be realised in practice, regardless of institutional resources. A nurse – or doctor, technician, porter, or admission clerk – always has a potential to extend a gesture that can affirm a patient's dignity. This gesture may be as little as a three-second pause, touching the patient and meeting their gaze. Such a gesture can be a powerful message, acknowledging what the ill person or family member is going through and affirming the nurse's presence, there for them. However inadequate institutional resources are, there are cracks in which one human can demonstrate recognition of the other's innate dignity as a fellow-human. No one is ever held hostage by institutional rules and resources.

Against that real potential for moral agency, nurses soon realise that their personal commitments to care are affected by institutional provision of resources. Being honest with oneself about what is and is not available helps a nurse not to set the bar too high on what dignity requires. Taking too much responsibility on oneself leads to a sense of failure, and burnout often follows. If Anne thinks she can spend her future career having time to invent creative ways to enable her patients to feel valued, she risks becoming embittered in most forms of healthcare work. If she then stays in nursing, she risks adapting by resignation: internalising an expectation that patients' dignity is a lost cause. Some of the nurses who complain to Elaine Maxwell may have crossed that threshold. Mary, who in Chapter 4 tells the story of treatment for breast cancer, offers a memorable description of such burned-out practitioners when she says: 'Health professionals are in a hurry; you can see it right away by the look in their eyes' (p. xx). Patients quickly learn to recognise that look, as they constantly examine those who come to examine them.

Another reason why nurses need to recognise what resources their institutional employers are failing to provide is that an important component of healthcare work – part of the job, both now and in the foreseeable future – is collective advocacy for the provision of what is necessary to respect the dignity of patients, starting with time and space. Clinical educators can find it very difficult to tell their students what is not well in the work they are embarking on. No one wants to hear that, so no one wants to say it. Yet, it is crucial to tell students that they are not only going to have to care for their patients; they are also going to have to negotiate and sometimes even militate for what they need in order to do that caring. Institutions, and those who regulate them, are not necessarily generous toward patients or staff; in most parts of the developed world, the opposite expectation is the norm. As grim as this reality may sound – as dark as it may seem to express it – it is a lapse of professional education to fail to inoculate students against the pressures they will face, and the corrosive effects those pressures can have on their personal and professional lives. Nurses who do not learn to be constructively critical of their institutions risk becoming destructively judgmental of their patients.

So much for underscoring what not only can but almost certainly will get in the way of nurses as they work, and often struggle, to effect in practice the ideals of dignity that are presented in the preceding chapters of this book. I now turn to why this struggle matters – why dignity matters so very much.

Again I quote Mary, describing being a patient with advancing breast cancer: 'sometimes, I felt I was treated as a diagnosis and a number in a row, while others managed to see me as a person' (p. xx). When I was receiving chemotherapy for cancer, a nurse who was speaking to my wife actually referred to me by tumour-type and room number; that label was how she knew me. I am sure the pressure was on her, and in those days cancer centres were far better funded per patient than they are today. But, as well as my wife and I realised what problems the nurses had in doing their work, we felt alienated – set apart, made to feel strange and estranged – as we struggled to do our work. Any patient's work is what Anatole Broyard, quoted by Oddgeir Synnes in Chapter 5, memorably described as avoiding becoming a 'diminished self' (p. xx). Mary poignantly rehearses the progressive diminishments that cancer effects in her shrinking life: losses of body parts and self-image; losses of potential for activity and the relationships that are part of those activities; and prospectively, the loss of life itself. Illness, by its nature, diminishes. Thus Broyard poses the great problem of being ill, a paradoxical dilemma: how not to experience one's self as diminished, even while one's life tangibly does diminish?

For many people, that dilemma opens into the sphere of the spiritual, which is given proper significance in Wilfred McSherry's chapter. But the restoration of dignity begins with simpler needs. Returning again to Mary's story, I value her description of the transition to palliative care (p. xx):

> When I first came in here (the curative unit), everything was hopeless; the pain overwhelmed me, and I did not want to live anymore. Here (in palliative care) it is absolutely fantastic: now I feel a new desire to live in the time I have left. One day, I was crying in bed; a nurse came in and just sat there until I had no more tears. It was of great importance.

I emphasise, the nurse just sat there. She had the resource of time, although I doubt it actually took so very long. Not always but often it takes remarkably little time to show another person that you are not rushing; you have time for them.

Mary does not specify more about what the palliative-care unit offers that was of such 'great importance' that it restored her will to live. I fill in her story with memories of when my mother, who was certain she was dying and seemed determined to die, was transferred from a curative unit to a palliative service. She lived for another year, time that included holding her great-grandchild and being with her extended family for another Christmas. The palliative unit provided quiet; it ended the constant needle sticks and other invasive procedures that, no matter how routine to nursing staff, had in their cumulative effect utterly sapped my mother's resolve; it provided a reasonably comfortable place for my father to sleep in the room with my mother; and it just slowed things down to my mother's pace. The spiritual could come later, or for some patients, maybe not. First, time and space.

Dignity is an expansive word, subsuming almost anything that people value about themselves and their lives. To some critics, that expansiveness renders the word vacuous, less than useful. I believe healthcare needs an expansive word as an ideal, a beacon in what can be the dark turbulence of healthcare practice. Or, to multiply metaphors, dignity is a true north to which one's moral compass can be reoriented, as the needle wavers between too many magnetic attractions.

One of the most important arguments in this book is that the dignity of the patient and the dignity of the healthcare professional inevitably exist in a symmetrical complementarity; each depends on the other. The final message is: preserve your dignity as a nurse and that hard-won disposition will enable you to know, as if by instinct, how to care for the dignity of your patients. Care for their dignity, and you will preserve your own.

Arthur W. Frank

Index